T0258887

Successful Models of Community Long Term Care Services for the Elderly

Successful Models of Community Long Term Care Services for the Elderly

Eloise H. P. Killeffer
Ruth Bennett
Editors

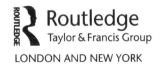

Routledge
Taylor & Francis Group

LONDON AND NEW YORK

First published 1990 by The Haworth Press, Inc.

Published 2018 by Routledge
2 Park Square, Milton Park, Abingdon, Oxon OX14 4RN
52 Vanderbilt Avenue, New York, NY 10017

Routledge is an imprint of the Taylor & Francis Group, an informa business

Copyright © 1990 Taylor & Francis

Successful Models of Community Long Term Care Services for the Elderly has also been published as *Physical & Occupational Therapy in Geriatrics*, Volume 8, Numbers 1/2 1989.

Library of Congress Cataloging-in-Publication Data

Successful models of community long term care services for the elderly / Eloise H.P. Killeffer, Ruth Bennett, editors.
    p. cm.
    Proceedings of a conference held in Nov. 1987 at the Columbia University School of Public Health and sponsored by its Division of Geriatrics and Gerontology.
    "Has also been published as Physical & occupational therapy in geriatrics, volume 8, numbers 1/2, 1989" — T.p. verso.
    Includes bibliographical references.
    ISBN 0-86656-987-1
    1. Aged — Long term care — Congresses. 2. Aged — Long term care — United States — Congresses. 3. Long-term care of the sick — Congresses. 4. Long-term care of the sick — United States — Congresses. I. Killeffer, Eloise H. P. II. Bennett, Ruth, 1933 — . III. Columbia University. Division of Geriatrics and Gerontology.
RA564.8.S83   1990
362.1'6 — dc20   89-29378
                                                                                              CIP

ISBN 13: 978-0-86656-987-3 (hbk)
ISBN 13: 978-1-138-88184-6 (pbk)

Successful Models of Community Long Term Care Services for the Elderly

CONTENTS

ERRATA

PAGES 37 AND 129: LTCPCC is an acronym for
Long Term Care Policy Coordinating Council,
not Committee or Counsel, as it appears on
these pages.

AMPLIFICATION AND CLARIFICATION
The conference upon which **Successful
Models**... is based was held in 1987, the
first year of operation of New York State's
Expanded In-home Services to the Elderly
Program (EISEP). Many of the presentations
focused on EISEP as it existed then; it has
since undergone changes which could not be
reflected in this book.

Readers wishing to know more about EISEP's
current operations are invited to contact
the Director of the EISEP Unit, New York
State Office for the Aging, 1 Empire State
Plaza, Albany, New York, 12223-0001,
telephone 518-474-8147.

ABOUT THE EDITORS

Eloise H. P. Killeffer, EdM, is Senior Research Scientist at the Columbia University Center for Geriatrics and Gerontology and Practicum Coordinator for the Division of Geriatrics and Gerontology, Columbia University School of Public Health. Her research activities have included cross-national studies of long term institutional care of the elderly, a national survey of innovative programs in long term care facilities for the elderly, and numerous evaluations of community-based service programs for the elderly.

She is a co-author of *Handbook of Innovative Programs for the Impaired Elderly* (Haworth Press, 1984) and editor of *Connections: An Adult Area Resource Directory* (United Way of New Canaan, Connecticut, 1989). She is a member of several task forces and advisory committees in the field of aging and belongs to both national and regional organizations on aging.

Ruth Bennett, PhD, is Director of Graduate Education of the Division of Geriatrics and Gerontology, Columbia University School of Public Health, Deputy Director of the Columbia University Center for Geriatrics and Gerontology, and Professor of Clinical Public Health (in the Center for Geriatrics and Gerontology and in Psychiatry) at Columbia University. Dr. Bennett is a member of numerous journal editorial staffs, task forces, and advisory boards.

She is co-author of *The Acting Out Elderly, Coordinated Service Delivery Systems for the Elderly, Handbook of Innovative Programs for the Impaired Elderly,* and *Continuing Care Retirement Communities: Political, Social and Financial Issues,* all published by The Haworth Press, and author of *Aging, Isolation and Resocialization* (Van Nostrand Reinhold, 1980).

In 1984, she received the Ollie Randall Award of the Northeastern Gerontological Society for her outstanding achievement and contributions in the field of gerontology. In 1984, she also received the Walter M. Beattie, Jr. Award for distinguished service in aging from the New York State Association of Gerontological Educators.

Preface

Communities are having to face the facts that they alone can determine the needs of their residents and they are best positioned to develop responses to those needs. Whether public monies are or are not available for long term care services for the elderly, their needs, precipitated by the demographic imperative, must be faced. While families can and do provide the bulk of care for the elderly, a number of factors preclude their providing care at all times for all of the elderly in any given community. Before relinquishing their obligations to protect and support all community residents of all ages, communities must look about, assess their resources and determine what they can do to maintain elderly residents in their homes and to preserve their dignity.

This book contains examples of successful community programs that have made use of a mix of public funding streams and private resources to provide long term care to elderly people residing in their own homes. These programs are considered successful for a number of reasons: each one has visible and outstanding leadership; each is financially sound, often using both public and private sources of funding; each is highly visible and accessible within the community; each has been ongoing for many years; and each incorporates many elements in order to provide for most of the needs of elderly residents as they "age in."

This is not to say that these programs were all instantly successful from the start: to the contrary, most of the authors of the following articles freely discuss the obstacles and barriers, bureaucratic and otherwise, with which they had to deal as their programs evolved and grew. Readers of this book may therefore learn from the experiences of others that successful community long term care services for the elderly are indeed possible, but not without great determina-

xiii

tion, resourcefulness and plain hard work. The editors and authors sincerely hope that this book may inspire others to achieve success in community programs for the elderly.

Eloise H. P. Killeffer, EdM
Ruth Bennett, PhD

Acknowledgements

The editors extend their greatest thanks to Susana Frisch, coordinator of the Administration on Aging grant that enabled the Division of Geriatrics and Gerontology in the Columbia University School of Public Health to establish its Master of Public Health (MPH) program with a specialization in long term care administration. Susana conceived the idea of the conference on which this book is based and worked tirelessly and unstintingly to coordinate every aspect of it (including the tape recording of all presentations, a brilliant stroke).

We also extend hearty thanks to all the presenters. Their collective wisdom, experience and insights, gathered between these two covers, affords a wealth of assistance and inspiration to those who would initiate new community long term care services for the elderly and improve existing ones.

Finally, the editors thank Melissa J. Solomon for her untiring labors at the word processor, transcribing tapes and converting endless pages of edited manuscript into finished copy.

Eloise H. P. Killeffer, EdM
Ruth Bennett, PhD
New York City
May 1989

xv

Introduction

Eloise H. P. Killeffer, EdM
Ruth Bennett, PhD

This volume is a compilation of articles based on the proceedings of a conference entitled "Successful Models of Community-Based Long Term Care for the Elderly" that was held at the Columbia University School of Public Health in November 1987 and was sponsored by their new Division of Geriatrics and Gerontology.

The purpose of the conference was to introduce students in the Division's Master of Public Health (MPH) with a specialization in long term care administration degree program to the concepts and issues surrounding the field of community-based long term care. The long term care administration program was developed under a 17-month grant from the Administration on Aging, which had as one of its major goals the development of training materials on community-based long term care. Important to this grant-funded program was the Advisory Committee that was set up to guide it (see listing of Advisory Committee members in the Appendices). This committee consisted of representatives of many organizations, agencies and professions in New York State and New York City who were (and still are) involved in all aspects of the development and delivery of community-based long term care services and programs for the elderly.

Because members of the Advisory Committee were very experienced and successful in their work on community-based long term care, Division faculty felt that students in the new program in long term care administration should be introduced to them and their work. The conference was seen as an ideal forum in which this introduction might occur. The assumption was that most, if not all, of the program's graduates would at some time in their careers work in the field of community-based long term care for the elderly.

While this field is still in its infancy, faculty felt that students would learn a great deal from those who are experienced in this field and would be inspired to continue to carry on the work about which they would learn in the conference.

The conference evaluations indicated that students and others who attended appreciated the opportunity to meet the speakers and to discuss the many topics and issues raised during the day's presentations. Many of the students were already interested in pursuing careers in community-based long term care and the talks and discussions encouraged them to continue this interest. To the extent that the conference fulfilled its aims, it was regarded as successful.

Successful Models
of Community-Based Long Term Care:
Implications for Graduate
Training Programs

Clifford Whitman, MSW

The Erie County (New York) Department of Senior Services began trying to coordinate long term care services in the late 1970s. Several attempts to establish a coordinating structure within the county government failed: the cause was not sufficiently popular politically at that time. The Department of Senior Services then conceived of an independent corporation; and in 1970, with the help of a Robert Wood Johnson Foundation grant, the Coordinated Care Management Corporation (CCMC) was created. CCMC brought together the public and private sectors: from the outset its board comprised county officials and presidents of non-profit service agencies (e.g., United Way and Catholic Charities). Its primary mission was to devise and implement a system of services for the frail elderly; that mission has been accomplished. With increased county funding, supplemented with additional foundation and community grants, its activities have expanded to include provision of case management services directly.

The Department's efforts to create CCMC were guided by a set of values deemed critical to the development of any long term care system; they are still important today. Foremost among these was consideration of the individual frail elder: he/she must have access to all needed services, and those services must be coordinated. Service delivery must be smooth and even.

Second was the need to create new coordinating mechanisms for both client service coordination (case management) and community agency coordination (systems development). The former would be accomplished by establishing case management in our neighborhood or cluster agencies, while the latter would be accomplished by creating the new corporation called CCMC.

Third was the need to integrate the health aspects of long term care with social support systems. CCMC emphasized the social support side of services since it was felt that the medical model had not worked and had proven too costly.

Fourth was the need to support a decentralized system of case management and services to take advantage of what was already in place and to minimize any disruption in the system. The point was to build on existing strengths, to enhance the contributions of service providers by coordinating their efforts and to see that there were no gaps across the whole service area.

Fifth was the belief that a neutral agency should be in charge of the overall systems development and should not offer services itself. This neutral group might be a separate new agency if it were feasible to create one; but since that is not usually the case, the Area Agency on Aging (AAA) might be the next most neutral existing entity. Neutrality was essential to avoid alienating conflicts of interest: e.g., placing the operation in the social service department would affront the health department and aging units; while locating it in the health department would engender other problems.

Sixth was the need for local determination of program design. Many counties were unhappy with never-ending state mandates.

Seventh was a belief that the system should operate on the neighborhood level where the community social support resources could be enlisted more easily to help. The underlying philosophy was that services are provided best by people who understand the community in which they live, people who know volunteer church groups and merchants and other community assets. Frail elders cannot be separated from their communities to be provided with costly services. CCMC instead subcontracted with neighborhood services and coordinated them. This reflected a belief in the public and private partnership. Community agencies that provide many of the local social supports had to be involved. Last was the need to give much support to the informal support systems of family and friends.

These underlying premises guided the development of CCMC in

Erie County. Its unique design and structure enabled it to function efficiently and to grow. The local Community Alternative System Agency (CASA) was placed in CCMC and eventually, it developed its own non-Medicaid case management system and home care program, through contract procedures and memoranda of understanding.

At the same time that CCMC was developing and expanding in its role in the early eighties, a series of demonstration projects emerged, all attempting to prove the value of community-wide systems development as well as the efficacy of case management as a mechanism of cost containment. The results of the case management effort were somewhat questionable regarding its cost saving qualities (only in those populations eligible for nursing homes were cost savings likely). Despite this, the conviction prevails that case management is the most humane way to deal with a very fragmented system of services to older persons.

Many of these projects have come and have gone, but in fact they did provide a number of lessons. The best thing that grew out of them was a commitment on the part of many states to develop and operate long term care programs: Oregon, Washington, Alabama, South Carolina, Wisconsin, Pennsylvania, New York and others became involved. The time had come for this activity to be fashionable, as each state struggled to control spiraling long term care costs. It was also during this time that it became obvious there was going to be little support for such efforts from the federal government: the states would have to take more leadership and funding responsibilities for long term care.

Communities and states devised various approaches to meeting the need for better long term care systems. This made searching for the best model to implement in one's community difficult and frustrating. The CASA notebook does provide a beginning conceptualization that is by no means exhaustive. These organizational models are (1) the single-entity model; (2) the single-entry/constituency-based client management model; and (3) the multiple-entry/constituency-based client management model.

The single-entity model vests system-wide and client management responsibilities in one organization. The same organization is also responsible for delivery of the services and controls much of the funding streams for the system. The best example of this model is Oregon, with both its Medicaid and non-Medicaid programs under the control of the State and Area Agencies on Aging. The Social Health Maintenance Organization (SHMO), the Long Term Home Health Care Program (Nursing Home without Walls, or Lombardi Bill Program) and the well-known On-Lok Program also represent this model. A similar approach here in New York State is the Broome County experience in Binghamton, N.Y., where all long term care, including the County CASA program, is operated by the Broome County Office for the Aging. Broome County took a very forward step by locating all the services of Medicaid nursing home placements in its Office for the Aging.

The single-entry/constituency-based client management system is another model that divides functions among client constituency groups. The systems-development function might be assumed by a new public or private entity or be assumed under an existing public agency. One agency performs all assessments and the clients are then referred to the appropriate agency for case management. A standard system of screening and case management can be accomplished through the use of common assessment and care planning instruments. There is concern here whether the case manager should not also be the assessor or vice-versa. There are also problems of efficiency and duplication in the model. Examples of these brokerage-type models are the Rochester ACCESS program and some of the channeling demonstration projects.

The multiple-entry/constituency-based client management model vests system-wide responsibilities in a separate entity. Client management and all its elements, including assessment, then are the responsibility of designated agencies, each serving a client constituency. Many people question the lack of a central point of intake in the design. Agency partiality to its own services is a danger in this situation and a strong performance monitoring system is needed. Erie County began with the multiple-entry model, in which case management is done through affiliated agencies, but moved toward the single-entity model: CCMC does some of its own assessment through the Heart Program, which it funds. This cooperative effort has enhanced understanding of the collaborative nature of CCMC.

These three models are by no means exhaustive. There are many variations of each of these models and some existing programs may even incorporate elements of each model. In fact, it appears that there is no one model that works in all communities. The best definition of the Utopian model is the one that works successfully in any given community, regardless of its configuration. Each community therefore may have its own unique model; this is confirmed by the present New York State approach: local autonomy is respected and each local community must work out, within certain limits, how they want such a program to be organized and to operate. Each program must take into consideration, therefore, the many crucial variables specific to the community it serves.

In reality, the success of any model depends on the processes by which it is established and maintained in any given community. Bringing all community service agencies together at the outset to plan and organize a long term care program may be difficult, but it is essential if the program is to succeed. Fordham University's Long Term Care Systems Management Training Project, under the direction of Jim McCormack, is a model well worth studying. It offers a Life Cycle Framework to understand better issues of structure and function across five management decision areas: technical, administrative, structural, political and financial. Each management decision area is broken down into five phases of the life cycle: preplanning, initiation, formalization, operation and fragmentation. A variety of issues then can be addressed within one or more appropriate phases. The fragmentation section is most interesting, for it highlights the need for on-going maintenance of the system. The elements of the system are always changing; people, politics, the organization and experience have shown that evolution of the system is a forgone conclusion.

By having a framework to deal with these necessary issues, one is better able to assess and analyze what will work in one's own community. This kind of conceptual framework may highlight the role that educational institutions can play in better preparing students for opportunities in community-based long term care programs. Not only are there opportunities to train large numbers of case managers and delivery system personnel that will be needed in these systems, but there is a need to help students understand elements involved in building and maintaining a coordinated system of long term care services. This is a new area that must be emphasized in light of the new movement throughout the country to reshape and improve the long term care system.

It must be recognized that some of the new programs have not yet been bureaucratized, and therefore it may not be easy to identify specific training requirements. It is essential to go out to the field and ask what is needed. It is necessary to involve committees, to do surveys, and even to study the backgrounds of those people presently working in the field. There is also an unusual opportunity to target different populations in training programs such as case managers and day care workers. The problem lies in the fact that this new area has not yet been standardized and therefore, it is difficult to be specific in the training. This will change in time as we witness more of the state standard-setting that is occurring already in order to assure the capacity of the long term care system within each state. The challenge is to bring together community agencies without sacrificing their autonomy, so they can provide all elderly, especially the frail and impaired, with appropriate and needed services in an effective, coordinated, systematic way. Training long term care professionals to understand the developmental process involved in establishing community-based long term care programs remains an educational priority.

PART I:
SERVICE PROVIDERS' ROLE
IN DEVELOPING SUCCESSFUL
MODELS OF COMMUNITY CARE

Introduction to Part I

The range of services provided to the elderly in the community is very broad, although the elderly are not mandated to use these services and often, even if they need them, will not have heard about them. Thus, the best advertisement for an organization or agency providing these services to the elderly in the community is a satisfied client.

The agencies described in this section have exceptionally good reputations in New York City and its environs. From them, students in the Division of Geriatrics and Gerontology are able to learn about state-of-the-art or best practices in administration and service delivery to the elderly in the community. These agencies have been around for some time and have experienced many of the hurdles and problems well-known throughout the field of community-based service delivery. The authors of the presentations below share some of the "tips" they have found useful in order to survive and flourish.

In addition, several of the authors discuss problems that have not been addressed to their satisfaction; it was profitable to conference attenders to have these issues aired.

9

Ellen Camerieri's chapter introduces this section on "Service Providers' Role in Developing Successful Models of Community Care." In her presentation on "Comprehensive Community Centers," she notes that senior centers are the easiest service for an elderly person to access because there are no eligibility criteria to satisfy other than age and city of residence. Once in such a center, the elderly person is made aware of most of the other services available to the elderly. Thus, ideally, the senior center is at the hub of the wheel of services that may be needed ultimately. Were there a community-based system in place, the senior center might be the perfect entry point into the system. Unfortunately, many elderly people do not become members of senior centers for all sorts of reasons. Therefore, they may remain uninformed about other services that are available until they reach a point of serious need. Under the best circumstances, it would be beneficial for all elderly to join senior centers, where they can not only learn about other services, but can socialize, engage in all kinds of activities, pursue all sorts of interests and participate in health promotion and illness prevention projects.

George Kaplan describes the New York City Home Attendant Program administered by the Jewish Association for Services for the Aged (JASA). In this chapter, he refers to the Extended In-Home Services for the Elderly Program (EISEP), which provides services to elderly persons just above the Medicaid level. He notes some of the problems encountered in administering this program. Lois Grau raises some problems in her discussion of "Home Care Services: Non-Professional Home Attendants."

Ralph Hall, in his chapter on "Day Care and the Continuum of Care," describes an adult day care program that is part of a major nursing home. The theme of nursing home-based community care is also addressed by Theresa Martico-Greenfield in "Nursing Home-Based Community Care." Institutions often are in a good position to share their resources with elderly persons who reside in the community. Thus, each nursing home can become a self-contained long term care system if it provides the full range of services along the continuum of care.

Igal Jellinek addresses the day-to-day problems encountered by community-based agencies trying the serve the elderly in an efficient and effective manner. Sometimes, this job can be accomplished only by coalescing with other agencies trying to serve the same population. His chapter on "Coalitions" discusses these and other related issues.

Douglas Holmes describes his research on "Special Populations" who may be underserved because of the lack of a true long term care system in any given community, city or state.

David Wilder describes his research on unmet needs of the community-based elderly. His chapter on "Filling the Housing and Service Gap" seems an appropriate way to end this section. Clearly, the community-based long term care system is in an embryonic stage — or, perhaps, in its infancy. All needs of all elderly people are not as yet being met. However, good starts have been made.

Comprehensive Senior Centers

Ellen Camerieri, CSW

Located in the Bronx, Riverdale Senior Services is a community-based multi-service program for the aging, like many others around the state and around the country. It is, for many older people, their first point of contact with the system, with the aging network—whatever it is called and whatever model is being used. Why would a center be the first point of contact? Primarily, because there is no assessment tool. A person must be sixty and live in New York City—it's that simple. He/she just walks in—if he/she likes it, he/she takes it; if he/she doesn't, he/she leaves. Nobody decides whether he/she is entitled to membership or not. In a sense, therefore, it's the most universally accessed form of service.

What are some of the distinguishing characteristics of a comprehensive senior center? "Center" here implies a much more total package than a meal and one activity a day. It is also much more than a nutrition site: rather, it is a full-service package. People come into a center at any point in the aging continuum. Riverdale Senior Services has members from sixty to ninety-six; indeed, there are more than a hundred people over ninety on the membership rolls, although not all of them currently come to the center. Recently, the center signed up a ninety-six-year-old gentleman who just walked in and decided that he may have reached the age at which the center might be of some service to him. Thus, the senior center is a very democratic agency. It touches people not only in different stages of aging but also at different levels of need. One could be sixty and in great need of medical and social services. Alternatively, one could be ninety-six and just want to join and participate in only one or two activities. Thus, there is a very wide variety of choice.

If the senior center is really part of the total aging services network, it is because it has developed strong linkages to the commu-

13

nity. Riverdale Senior Services is very fortunate because its board is a part of the local community. In many ways, Riverdale is more of a small town than a New York City neighborhood, in the sense that most people think of New York City neighborhoods; and the board is local, committed and talented. The agency grew out of a perceived need in the community and was tailored over the years to meet the changing needs that have been expressed within the community.

Riverdale Senior Services has many points of contact with the larger service system, the more formalized aging network. First is strong contacts with metropolitan New York Schools. Students from Columbia University's Schools of Public Health and Dentistry and the Programs in Occupational Therapy pursue geriatric specializations through placements at the center. Student nurses from Mt. St. Vincent College receive team training with community elderly. This exposure helps combat the sick role myths about the elderly, for the students see that not all elderly are so deteriorated that they must be institutionalized, in either hospitals or nursing homes. Indeed, many of the people who are coming to centers today would have been in institutions in prior years.

What does this say for today's senior centers? It says that they have to do an incredible stretch to serve recent retirees who are just looking for a way to maintain their ego identities with some useful, meaningful involvement, as well as the growing numbers of frail elderly, the newly-widowed, and the almost-infirm and, in some cases, even Alzheimer's patients. Many elderly coming to the center need more care than we can offer, but if they had not come to the senior center, they would not later be referred to the services and programs they need. Thus, senior centers have to know all the resources and have good connections with them. They must not be proprietary; they must want to get elderly people to the services that will benefit them, which is not always where we would like to have them.

Riverdale Senior Services cooperates with many of the resources in New York City, such as the Hunter-Brookdale program which provides trained Medicare volunteers. This is necessary because many Medicare recipients simply pile up bills and never seek reimbursement, because it is all just too confusing. Even when a statement says "this is not a bill," many elderly pay it anyway. Trained volunteers are invaluable resources in this regard. The social worker at Riverdale Senior Services facilitates Medicaid applications for elderly attenders. Trained by the New York City Department of Social Services, she is authorized to pre-certify, thus easing the initial stages of entry into that system. Final certification must be done at the Social Services Office, however. These are all very acceptable and useful services for recent retirees who want to continue to do something, who want to be affiliated with the aging network — but not too affiliated, because they're not too aged yet.

All of the services provided by Riverdale Senior Services stretch a very small staff, even though the center is considered to have a good staffing model: a director who is a social worker; an assistant director, also a social worker, who does the social service supervision and the student supervision; and a program director who puts together a package that goes from art to yoga, and that includes many volunteers. Many members themselves are volunteers: e.g., a seventy-five-year-old yoga instructor who appeared in the Riverdale Press standing on his head. Riverdale Senior Services has wonderful resources, and it tries to capitalize on them. But there are two hundred people a day on the premises. Visitors from nursing homes have inquired about the staffing patterns, and they are amazed to learn that it consists mostly of preprofessionals and support staff. This minimal staffing has one advantage, however: it compels the center to draw upon the people themselves and their relatives and friends and to turn to the community for support.

However, the concept of multi-service senior centers has gone just about as far as it is going to go without additional overhead resources. New service packages are made available offering money, e.g., for transportation of volunteers, but without allowance for more staffing; and centers are expected to run this little transportation program for a thousand people. Or, an Alzheimer's respite program may be offered, but with staff only one day a week. Riverdale Senior Services rarely declines such opportunities, but finding funds to participate in these programs is increasingly difficult. So it is that multi-service senior centers must demand adequate funding to support the variety of programs needed to serve their members appropriately and well. Senior centers also have to fight to retain those characteristics that have made aging services so gratifying over the years — the mix of people: the ethnic mix, the income mix, the age mix. While increased professionalization is laudable, increased bureaucratization is deplorable. Is a twenty-page EISEP assessment tool really necessary for somebody who needs four or eight or twelve hours of home care a week? Is the overhead incurred in centralizing something like this justified? Is the machinery going to outpace the service? There is no easy answer to this one, because things cannot be done the way they used to be, in terms of the numbers, the needs, the increased lifespan, and not just the increased numbers, but the increased frailty. But the EISEP partnership has got to be more than just a paper partnership; what is occurring with the area agency in this area is much more of a paper than a real partnership. This could be extremely destructive if it does not change. Although this may be viewed, generally speaking, as resistance to change or intransigence, perhaps it is just a different perception of what the needs are and how they can be met. There must be a marriage, and there must be a dialogue. Opportunities such as this conference give us some hope for a happy marriage.

New York City Home Attendant Program

George Kaplan

The Jewish Association for Services for the Aged (JASA), based in New York City and covering Nassau and Suffolk counties as well, is a multi-purpose social service agency and an affiliate of the Federation of Jewish Philanthropies. JASA provides a variety of services, including case work, group work, housing, legal services, nutrition and transportation. Another service offered by JASA is home care, provided through three subsidiary corporations with two contracts, one from the Human Resources Administration and one from the New York City Department for the Aging. This is the new EISEP: Expanded In-Home Services for the Elderly Program. This presentation concerns the home attendant program, JASA's role in it and some of their experiences with it.

EISEP evolved from a rather informal housekeeping/homemaking program, based at Montefiore Hospital, that existed even before Medicaid. In the early 1970s, Medicaid began paying for these services, but it soon became apparent that exceptions to their existing policies were becoming necessary more and more frequently. That is, many elderly people (e.g., those just discharged from hospitals) needed more housekeeping/homemaking services than Medicaid allowed, so waivers were granted and these elderly were given Medicaid funds to purchase the additional services privately. Thus for some six or seven years, thousands of two-party checks (in the names of both client and home attendant) were issued by New York City so that additional needed services could be obtained. The problems associated with this system were numerous and predictable: checks were issued to incorrect names; there was no supervision of services; extortion was practiced by both clients and home attendants. In 1980, after several years of false starts, New York City decided to vendorize its program: contracts were drawn up with some 37 various agencies (social services and health, both local and city wide) to provide housekeeping/homemaking services to an estimated 15,000 clients.

Today, there are 60 agencies providing these services to some 35,000 clients through EISEP. In 1987 this represented about 93 million hours of service at a cost of $700 million. JASA holds two of these contracts; its program provides weekly services to about 1,600 clients—some 3.5 million hours of service per year, with an annual budget of $12 million. The home attendant program is growing in size about 8% annually and counting.

New York State's contribution to the cost of this program has decreased from 25% to 10%, thereby shifting a greater share of the burden to New York City, which is itself under great pressure to reduce Medicaid costs. Approximately 90% of all Medicaid dollars spent on long term care are consumed in New York City, as are about 70% of all federal funds supporting home care. The need to contain these costs has led to inevitable conflicts: when funds are limited and service needs keep growing with the increased elderly population, what trade-offs can be made? Certainly, there are no easy answers.

In the meantime, JASA's home attendant program operates under strict fiscal controls: every expenditure from salaries to pencils is regulated by New York City's Medicaid office. In an effort to elevate home attendant services from the perceived position of "home care's stepchildren," the 60 EISEP agencies have organized into a Home Care Council; dues paid by member agencies support an office and a salaried executive director. The Council has thus become an agent of its members and can negotiate with New York City and New York State about fiscal constraints.

Although EISEP provides vital services to thousands of elderly people, its continued existence depends on more than the determination and political power of the 60 home attendant service agencies and their Council. The voters must take a more active role in communicating to their elected officials that home attendant services for the impaired elderly must continue to receive priority. Maintaining the elderly at home and thereby avoiding, or at least deferring, institutionalization should be more than a strictly economic consideration: humanitarian concerns are at issue as well.

Home Care Services:
Non-Professional Home Attendants

Lois Grau, PhD

The preceding papers have addressed a variety of what seem to be nearly ideal models, as well as the critical issue of how one matches a model to a specific community. Unfortunately, the reality in this country is that most people do not have access to any of these models—ideal or close to ideal. This is particularly true with respect to non-professional home care (not a particularly good term, but it covers the gamut of titles involved in this particular type of service delivery). There is not any kind of model for the delivery of non-professional care, because this country does not have a national health care policy for community care. What it does have are frail elderly with a variety of disabilities and needs. There are various funding streams, such as Title III of the Older Americans Act, Title XX of the Social Security Act and Medicaid and Medicare of that act. There is a whole range of job titles, from home health aid to home attendant to personal attendant, then to personal care worker to chore worker, all of which are a direct result of the particular type of funding stream that supports that particular worker and program. And there is a range of organizations that deliver non-professional care, including both proprietary and not-for-profit community home care agencies, proprietary and not-for-profit hospitals, county and local government agencies, and nursing homes which are becoming a part of this service as well.

The picture is further complicated by the fact that some types of non-professional home care fall under the rubric of the "medical" model, whereas others fall under the "social" model. Very few of these home care programs are of the type that would warrant the title "medical-social," (see "Day Care and the Continuum of Care" by Ralph E. Hall in this collection); that may be a more ideal

19

variety of theoretical context for the delivery of services. In addition to those various factors that must be dealt with, it is also true that the delivery of non-professional care varies in terms of the context of the service. In some situations it is delivered with complete autonomy (using that word not in an ideal sense, but in a real sense): there are no controls whatsoever. Families can and do hire workers through the newspaper or through various types of church and information sources, and they are completely on their own. In other programs, a service is provided through an agency, but with relatively little contact with any other type of professional worker. In the state of California, workers in the welfare program in fact cannot even get a car loan through a bank because their employer is the person for whom they are caring. Thus there are many, many problems not only in the nature of the work and the model in which it resides, but also in the specific organizational context from which it comes.

The type of program or type of non-professional service an older person receives is the result of a multitude of factors. The most important are probably the physical health status of the individual with respect to illness acuity; their financial status in terms of ability to pay out of pocket for services and entitlement to means-tested programs; their geographic residence with respect to service availability and the presence and tenacity of someone to access the system for them; and luck with respect to all of the above. What then is the best or ideal model of care? The answer seems to be a model whose program is available, accessible, coordinated, monitored and flexible. It also assumes that a service should not be provided in isolation, but rather as a part of a larger package, which draws variously on other services as they are needed over time. Thus, while it may be that non-professional home care is the primary type of care needed, it should not be left to run off on its own. There has to be some kind of overview, some kind of monitoring to be sure that it doesn't become an entity unto itself.

The closest approximations to ideal models of care are many of those that have been described in other presentations, including some of the larger demonstration projects such as Triage and Channeling. These projects are characterized by case management approaches and many of them are driven by cost-containment motives (e.g., the impact of formal community care on the provision of informal family care and the use of costly health services such as nursing home care and hospital care). However, most of these programs tend to be short-lived. Fortunately, that tends not to be as true in New York State as in other parts of the country. One reason we do not see the replication of such demonstration projects is that evaluation study after evaluation study failed to demonstrate that this type of formal community care is cost-effective in terms of reducing the use of costly health care services. That orientation to evaluation is something that should be questioned. The fact that we have not been able to demonstrate that such programs as Triage and Channeling save a lot of money may be why non-professional community workers, by far the least expensive form of community home care, often operate in relative isolation. It is still not cheap, but it is far less costly than the $40.00 to $60.00 an hour cost of sending a nurse or another professional into the home. In many programs, including the home attendant program in New York City, there is great variety with respect to the extent of involvement of nurses and social workers in training, supervision and monitoring of care. Some agencies attempt to do this and do it very well, whereas in others, home care workers will talk with the supervisor only when they feel they have a problem and happen to give them a call.

The challenge now is implementation of a more ideal model of care that includes non-professional care. The critical need to look not only at the client assessment but also community assessment in terms of matching models to community needs has been discussed elsewhere. It is intriguing that the work that Jim McCormack (at Fordham) and others are doing is finally receiving some kind of attention: ten years ago, community assessment was the byword in public health, only to be replaced by quality assurance, then cost-effectiveness, then cost-containment. Finally, community assessment is again in vogue.

The need now is to prepare people with creative, open minds, as well as those with informed and realistic minds. The problems in long term care are incredibly complex and must be attacked at many different levels. One of them is the national level: while it is critical to train people to do hands-on provision of service at the local level, it is necessary to think beyond trying to manipulate the pieces of the current system and to consider what can be done at a higher level to streamline both resource channels and management approaches. Those directly involved in home care may not comprehend how bureaucratized it has become, but those outside the system (e.g., a researcher trying to draw a sample) are very struck by it. One must ask questions about the costs of the multiple and sometimes overlapping systems that have developed, not only in terms of their effectiveness with respect to various kinds of outcomes but also in terms of their humaneness with respect to managers and clients alike. Another crucial issue is the validity of distinguishing social from medical care models for the delivery of non-professional services. This problem is not new: the tension between the two approaches is well-known, as is the need to bring them together. However, the reality is that funding streams totally determine what kind of orientation a program will take, even though the actual work of the non-professional home attendant may not differ perceptibly from that of her professional counterpart.

It is essential to consider whether elderly clients should be differentiated by their need for skilled care (e.g., Medicare entitlement criteria) versus unskilled care, with respect to the delivery of non-professional services. If that classification is valid, one might then ask why people who are classified as ''skilled'' receive fewer hours of non-professional care than those in the Medicaid program who are classified as ''unskilled.'' Further, it is important to focus on training and supervision of non-professional workers. The evening news suggests that this country has headed into the scandals of the 1980s—homecare abuses (compared to the nursing home scandals of the seventies), which are a strong argument for the training of non-professionals. They need to know how to lift, to cook, to clean. There is a call now from AARP to recognize the need for non-professionals to perform more acute kinds of intervention, such as respirator care and parenteral feeding. All of that is important; no one would deny that. But the reality for a non-professional home care worker and her client is that this is a psycho-social relationship at heart. It has to do with two people together in somebody's home over time, often twenty-four hours a day. Not accepting that is putting heads in the sand. Reported scandals attest to the need to have some kind of mechanism to recognize, to train, and to monitor the nature of the relationship that exists between clients and their workers to prevent these sorts of abuses. It should be noted, however, that the abuses are not just one way. Home care workers are abused by elderly clients and their families. In fact, a recent study by the author of 600 home care workers has revealed a plethora of improprieties: that telephone numbers were disconnected, people had moved, clients didn't exist. The study also elicited horror stories from home care workers, such as this response to the interviewer's question, "How do you feel about your job?"

> Well, I'll tell you what my job is like. About a month ago I went to this home for the first time, and there was an old lady, and I liked her. And the daughter was there, and the daughter was nice, and boy they make me feel so good, so needed. The place was really in bad shape: there were roaches. I didn't know that I wanted to work there, but I thought she was such a nice lady, and that I'd really get the place cleaned up. They showed me my room, and it really wasn't a room, it was just a closet area with just a piece of material for privacy, and there was only a mattress on the floor. But you know that's alright. It's a seven-day, twenty-four hour a day job, I'll take it. All of a sudden by the next week, nobody was real grateful to have me around. They took me for granted. And by the third week, the daughter was asking me to do her laundry. And so forth and so on. Well finally, I quit last week. I don't have any money, but I've got my bed!

It is obvious that attention must be paid not just to the service needs of the client, but to the interaction of the client with worker, so informed decisions can be made whether to continue non-professional home care. Perhaps it is not appropriate: many of the clients in the Medicaid program are incredibly difficult to care for, and if the safety of the home care worker is in jeopardy, alternatives must be sought.

There is considerable debate about the general effectiveness of formal community-based care programs in reducing the use of hospitals and nursing homes by the elderly. While cost-effectiveness and cost-containment are legitimate concerns, they should not be the sole basis for making decisions about the kinds of services the elderly receive and from whom. However, in considering models of community care, serious attention must be given to the interplay of factors that influence choices (and frequently dictate them): the elderly's economic status, the availability and intensity of informal caregiving resources, personal values and preferences, local hospital and nursing home occupancy rates and cultural aspects such as intergenerational reciprocity and responsibility. In short, the problem is less that of knowing what a good or ideal model of care looks like than of arguing its value to multiple and sometimes competing segments of society. Home care should not be a substitute for other kinds of care, but rather one element of a total system of services.

Day Care and the Continuum of Care

Ralph E. Hall, MA

Since 1977, Morningside House, located in the Bronx, New York, has been providing a program of services specifically designed to serve the "ambulatory confused resident"—now usually identified as the individual with Alzheimer's disease. Morningside House and its affiliate, Aging in America, also serve as the EISEP agency for Community Districts 11 and 12 in the Bronx. In 1986 this program was expanded to include a community-based day care program for clients with dementia. This program is discussed here. However, to understand the significance of the rapidly-developing number of day care centers across this country and this state, it is important to view the day care center as part of a larger continuum of care.

GENERALIZED STATEMENTS ABOUT DAY CARE PROGRAMS

There are many discussions both within New York State and across the country regarding the different models of day care. The variety of these models include

1. The Medical Model
2. The Social-Medical Model
3. The Continuum of Care Model
4. The Volunteer Social Model

Although these titles are not used by all day care systems, any variants do not change perceptibly the definition of each model:

1. The *Medical Model* often accents rehabilitation by employing the skills of physicians, nurses and therapists in addressing the needs of patients/clients who have experienced a traumatic episode

25

which has resulted in limiting physical and mental capabilities. The length of stay of this model may be shorter than other models.

2. The *Social-Medical Model*, the model used at Morningside House, is guided by professional oversight with an organizational structure often linked to other medical care providers. The clients may need both social and medical services, and rehabilitation with discharge may not be a feasible alternative. Clients usually have a longer length of stay in this model.

3. The *Continuum of Care Model*, to which Morningside House hopes to move very shortly, provides within the same general area, day care programs that combine the efforts of the first two models with that of the fourth. An individual may enter this program of continuity as a member of the social day care program with no medical requirements. If the client's status changes, he/she can slowly progress to a more comprehensive program. This seems to be the more appropriate model, both in terms of dollars and cents and in terms of patient/client need.

4. The *Volunteer Social Model* appears to be a slightly more structured senior center with an accent on recreational, social and emotional support to the clients. Although Morningside House has significant experience with directing a senior center of about 1,000 members, it has no experience in this model of day care program.

Nancy Mace, author of *The 36-Hour Day*, has often remarked that as she travels across the country, she has difficulty distinguishing between the clients in medical models and the clients in social models. She suspects, probably with reason, that in many locations, the real difference between the two models may be the funding and only the funding.

MORNINGSIDE HOUSE ALZHEIMER'S DAY CARE PROGRAM

Morningside House currently operates a State-approved, Non-Occupant Day Care Program which, according to State Code, must be operated as part of a State-approved program (in this case Morningside House, a skilled nursing facility). This approach entitles clients to Medicaid support as long as the program is operated within the guidelines of the State.

The program now serves 25 clients a day, five days a week. Rarely are there fewer; in fact, there is a very long waiting list at present. State approval has been requested to expand to 35 clients for seven days a week. Indications are favorable that this will be approved due to the nature of the special clients served by this program.

The program includes transportation, noon-time meal, family support and medical oversight, with an accent on social-recreational-emotional support. Staff consists of the director, one full-time nurse, one full-time nurse's aide, three recreational therapists (including one music therapist), a part-time social worker, an office manager and the professional back-up of the team at Morningside House. Staff would increase as needed, with State approval for expansion.

All clients admitted to the program must have a diagnosis of dementia. Based on observation of other programs, this factor is probably the most important one in understanding the need for the medical oversight and supervision. It is very likely that the clients served within this program would not do well without this professional oversight. This is not to say that dementia patients would not do well in other programs; rather, patients in this particular program need the medical oversight in order to make the program truly worthwhile.

The Experience of Morningside House with Its Day Care Program

The model has surpassed the highest expectations of everyone at Morningside House. While a major fear in opening a new program is the cost associated with a long-term start-up period, Morningside House was able to reach maximum census within five months. Ongoing evaluation of client satisfaction (including families) has been very positive.

Approximately 95% of the program's clients are Medicaid recipients. Earlier research by Morningside House suggested that there might be a problem in attracting Medicaid-approved individuals. This has not eventuated. Another potential obstacle to the success of Medicaid-supported programs — working with the New York

City Medicaid office—was avoided through the development of a liaison with the local Bronx Medicaid office. This tremendous cooperation has enabled the Morningside House Day Care Program to process its eligible clients rapidly into the Medicaid system.

Many day care programs choose a nurse as the director. Morningside House chose instead a member of its team who had successfully demonstrated management and care abilities as Director of Recreational Therapy there. This has proven to be a very appropriate decision, as the program has developed with a splendid balance of social and medical considerations. The full-time Medical Director at Morningside House does provide medical guidance to the program, but clients retain their private physicians. (In contrast, in the Skilled Nursing Facility, only employed medical staff may serve as primary physicians.) Financially, the program has supported itself very well. Indeed, there is concern that the State may request that some funds be returned.

System Integration

The director of the day care program reports to the Administrator of Morningside House. All the staff listed above report directly to the director, with the exception of the social worker, who is part of the Morningside House Social Work Department. Development, long-range planning and financial management for the Alzheimer's Day Care Program are integrated into the management of the Morningside House-Aging In America family.

THE FUTURE OF THE DAY CARE PROGRAM AT MORNINGSIDE HOUSE

As noted earlier, the program is moving to the Continuum of Care Model, based on expectations of improvement in the system. This new model will include

1. An Alzheimer's home care program, managed as a component of the day care program, that will include respite services. (State approval must be sought for this added program through submission of a Certificate of Need.) This combination of home care and day

care is unusual, but Morningside House believes such a dual program best serves the needs of its clients.

2. A social day care program that will be operated physically in space adjacent to the current program. Some of the programming will actually be the same for both groups of clients. The major distinction between the two client populations would be their medical needs: those with higher requirements would remain in the existing model, with reimbursement primarily through State funds. Those individuals with dementia who are experiencing little or no medical problems would be supported by the new program on a fee-for-services basis. Unfortunately, to keep the expenses reasonable, transportation may not be possible in the new model.

3. A new case management system to support clients across all programs at Morningside House. When an individual seeks support from either Morningside House or an agency with which it contracts, it will be possible to address a full range of needs, including day care, home care, meals-on-wheels, spouse support, transportation and medical services. This client-focused case management will improve the services provided.

4. The continuation of inpatient services at Morningside House, but with changes as well. Successes with the non-resident day-care program have led to implementation of a resident day care program for twenty-four residents, to be operated seven days a week, from 10:00 a.m. to 4:00 p.m. within Morningside House. It will operate the same as the day care program described above, except that these clients will return to their rooms within Morningside House each night.

The Future Managers of Day Care Programs

The best experience for potential managers in this area is a field experience. As an organization that believes the best managers are those who have actual client-support relationships, Morningside House feels that students could obtain this experience in a variety of ways within the day care setting. The models attached to a continuum of services probably provide better career opportunities for entry-level managers. The continuum of care model at Morningside House represents a new and developing service model. However, the skills being taught now to those preparing to work with geriatric clients are appropriate for all models discussed in this paper. Perhaps there should be a slightly stronger emphasis upon case management with a client focus, coupled with a broader understanding of continuum of care service planning, in order to support students in their new endeavors.

Nursing Home-Based Community Care

Theresa Martico-Greenfield, MPH

HISTORY OF HOME CARE AT JHHA

As early as the 1930s, the Jewish Home and Hospital for Aged (JHHA) was providing for the needs of the elderly at home. It was recognized then that those on the waiting list for admission often needed support, and when someone was being admitted to the home, there frequently was a spouse, sibling or other family member who also needed support and assistance to remain in the community. So JHHA began to provide home care services for this purpose well before they were established as part of care for the aged.

Making a leap of some 40 years, JHHA — now a 1,326-bed nursing home — is providing a range of community-based services at its campuses in Manhattan and the Bronx to as many or more people as receive inpatient services — that means more than 1,300 people in communities throughout those two boroughs.

JHHA'S CONTINUUM OF COMMUNITY-BASED CARE

The range of community-based services being provided by the home includes

1. A social work outreach program called Geriatric Outreach (GO) that provides socialization, regular social work contact, telephone reassurance, crisis intervention, psychiatric consultation and case management as needed; and is targeted to frail elderly on the Upper West Side of Manhattan who have few or no informal supports;

2. A medical-model geriatric day center and a geriatric day cen-

31

ter for the blind and visually impaired, a collaborative program with the Jewish Guild for the Blind;

3. Senior housing at various levels — Kaufmann Residence for totally independent living; Kittay House, a 300-unit apartment house for the "well elderly," with meals and housekeeping; and enriched housing for congregate living with social services, housekeeping services and one congregate meal daily;

4. Home health care, through the Long Term Home Health Care or Lombardi "Nursing Home without Walls" Program for those with chronic needs; and through the recently-approved certified home health agency, which provides acute home care services;

5. A new follow-up service for residents discharged from the short term intensive rehabilitation unit, including social service linkage, referral, revision of care plans and, as needed, case management for those discharged residents;

6. A fledgling program called Geriatric Counseling that includes psychosocial assessments, referral and family and individual counseling focused on the struggles and conflicts associated with caring for the elderly person;

7. Approval as a Comprehensive Outpatient Rehabilitation Facility (CORF), to provide restorative rehabilitation and social work services to elderly living in the community; and

8. An innovative off-site program at the Penn South Housing Cooperative, in collaboration with Self-Help and the Educational Alliance, to provide direct social work service to frail elderly Penn South cooperators interested in exploring JHHA's range of community programs as well as discussing their reactions to the idea of nursing home placement.

POSITIVES AND NEGATIVES
OF JHHA'S COMMUNITY CARE MODEL

JHHA's continuum of community-based care model has both positive and negative features. Perhaps most positive is the clients' connection to JHHA. From this connection, no matter what the program or service involved, comes trust: trust that JHHA will provide

for changing needs; that it will be a resource; that if institutionalization becomes appropriate and/or preferable, the facility will make
every effort to have the elderly person admitted there. Through this
connection to JHHA, clients begin to view the nursing home not as
a place to be feared, but as a place that encourages their independence and provides resources to assist them in remaining independent.

From the perspective of each community program, another positive aspect is the relative ease with which linkages can be made to
other JHHA programs. Whether for a new referral or a current client, program staff have easy access to each other and can develop a
plan of care that suits the client's needs.

There are a few negatives to consider, however. One is funding
for those programs that are badly needed but are not reimbursable.
For JHHA, these include Geriatric Outreach, Penn South off-site
services and the follow-up program for residents discharged from
the rehabilitation unit. In an era of RUGs reimbursement, the search
for outside funding sources has intensified. Other programs receiving government subsidy or reimbursement struggle to break even
because the rates allowed do not usually meet operating costs — yet
these programs are vital resources for the elderly at a time when
discharge from hospitals is quicker, no new nursing home beds are
being built and home care is struggling to expand to keep up with
needs.

Another negative is that nursing home-based community programs often lead to unrealistic expectations on the part of clients
and staff. For example, JHHA cannot provide primary or emergency medical care or on-call social service staff to its community
clients because it does not have a certificate to operate an outpatient
department. However, when a community client is in the throes of a
medical emergency, JHHA is often called, especially when it is that
client's only support in the community. Clients expect a nurse, doc-
tor and/or social worker to go to their aid no matter how frequently
or persistently they may have been told when they became clients
that JHHA cannot provide emergency medical services. Staff who
receive these calls — switchboard operators, social workers, administrators — also often expect to be able to offer assistance beyond

calling 911 for the client. Thus, JHHA often does respond even though to do so stretches its resources beyond their realistic limits. The parameters of JHHA as a resource are difficult to set and to stick to, and it is even more difficult to limit expectations.

INTERFACING

Every program interfaces with the larger service delivery system, including hospital admitting departments and discharge planners; senior housing providers and landlords; home care providers, public and private; senior centers and day care programs; entitlement programs; community physicians; regulators; community coalitions or provider agencies; volunteers; and the New York City Department for the Aging. Each component of the system can, at one time or another, provide vital information about or for a client or provide essential services for a client. Together, the programs at JHHA work with these sources to meet most appropriately the needs of clients. This is very difficult given the extreme fragmentation of services: even within types of service, like home care or day care, there is fragmentation because of regulations, reimbursement mechanisms and agency policies. Often, clients receive services from a number of agencies because of the way services are "organized," and no one is responsible overall for seeing that the care is received or for ensuring that services are not duplicated.

IMPLICATIONS

This implies that there is need to develop a system in which it is possible for services to be rendered in a rational manner so that all who need services can receive them: a system in which regulatory and reimbursement decisions are made with great forethought about, and planning for, the impact these decisions will have on other parts of the service delivery system. It also implies that community service providers and consumers need to build coalitions and to collaborate on working toward a more cohesive system.

TRAINING STUDENTS

Students can be involved in developing nursing home-based community programs first by realizing that while there are nursing homes that continue to provide inadequate care, there are many high-quality nursing homes with a commitment to residents, to communities and to learning. Students need to understand how the population served on an inpatient basis by nursing homes has changed. Similarly, they need to see how the nursing homes' expertise in having cared for these differing elderly populations can be used to develop ways of maintaining these aged in their communities. An important component of good nursing home care is the interdisciplinary care team. Students should have early and repeated opportunities to work with students in other disciplines to problem-solve and prepare practical projects or papers. Practicum and residency curricula should be designed to insure that students have these experiences in the agency setting. The nursing home, in collaboration with university programs, can serve as a central point for education in community-based long term care administration.

The Role of Community-Based Coalitions

Igal Jellinek

This presentation focuses on several issues that can be addressed best by coalitions. The examples here are drawn from several coalitions with which the author has been associated in New York City. It is clear that services and resources needed by the elderly as well as those who work with them cannot be obtained easily by one agency working alone. A coalition of all or most agencies serving the elderly in any given community can do better than any one agency in relation to advocacy, visibility, funding and planning. Below are some examples based on the author's own experience with coalitions.

ADVOCACY FOR ADULT DAY CARE

Those working with the elderly have long recognized the need for adult day care and have joined in coalitions to advocate for it. Dr. Barry Gurland and others at the Columbia University Center for Geriatrics and Gerontology conducted a study of adult day care centers in New York State, focusing mainly on health-related day care. In addition, New York Governor Mario Cuomo issued a report containing a blueprint of what elderly day care should be, which was put out by the Long Term Care Policy Coordinating Council (LTCPCC, referred to by John Wren, pp. 129-133). They recognized the need for socialization, transportation and health services. They noted also that the constituency for the mentally retarded and developmentally disabled had succeeded in setting up some excellent day care programs in New York State. Thus, these reports gave those working with the elderly some reference points.

As president of the Adult Day Care Committee of Greater New York and as treasurer of the Day Care Committee, both interagency

37

coalitions, the author met two years ago with LTCPCC in Albany. This meeting was nothing less than abysmal because no one talked to each other: the Health Department people looked only at health; the Office of Mental Health people looked only at mental health. The idea of interdisciplinary collaboration seemed not to have reached them. Fortunately, the two interagency coalitions represented by the author stood together and did not falter under the barrage of questions thrown at them. This meeting led to some changes and two years later, a policy statement signed by Governor Cuomo was presented at an adult day care conference attended by the author and others at today's conference.

It is important when advocating to be well-informed and to stand one's ground. It is equally important to know what one wants and why. An illustration from another meeting with Governor Cuomo shows how decisions can be made in the absence of a firm position. In 1986, he asked, "Do you want the SSI pass-through or do you want the prescription drug bill?" People were not prepared to answer that question and said, "That's your decision. That's what we pay you for and that is what you got elected for." That was the wrong response. Those working with the elderly must be prepared to answer such questions by having facts on what is needed and wanted by their elderly constituencies. Therefore, coalitions must include groups that can anticipate such questions and get answers quickly.

Another illustration of coalition development concerns monitoring and responding to the several governmental and decision-making bodies that affect a particular group of service providers: agencies receiving contracts from New York City. In 1987, a new policy called the welfare-to-work initiative was created by the Board of Estimate for all agencies receiving city contracts. In response, a number of these agencies, all large, including the Council of Senior Centers and Services (which represents 242 agencies that contract with the New York City Department for the Aging and the Senior Center Division of the New York City Human Resources Administration [HRA]), Child Care Inc., the Day Care Council and others formed an ad hoc group that decided to call itself a coalition. Such coalitions are very effective when they respond immediately to a government initiative. In fact, coalitions exist because of government: governments see things from very different perspectives and it is essential to keep them honest. They must be told when policies have adverse effects and when they will work.

VISIBILITY

Groups with the same or similar interests may coexist in a community without knowing about each other and without knowing how they affect one another. In the 1970s, the author headed a multi-service agency that provided social day care to the elderly. It ran the second-largest transportation program in New York City and its senior center served a minority population (about 80% of its members were Hispanic).

Columbia University and the Presbyterian Hospital were about five blocks away. At that time, the Center for Geriatrics and Gerontology was formed at the Columbia University Medical Center. The author wondered how his agency and the University might work together. People in the community were saying, "They're researchers. How can that be turned into services?" The author believed then, and still believes, that this kind of collaboration is a challenge that agencies must pursue and foster. Thus the author's agency was able to enlist the help of Patricia Miller and Dr. Barbara Neuhaus of the Program in Occupational Therapy at Columbia: they obtained a grant to support students to work with the center's elderly clients. That helped the center take over a Self-Help-sponsored program that was attenuating for lack of funds: a social day care program for the frail elderly which was then consolidated into the senior center. Thus, the center gave visibility to the OT training program and OT gave visibility to the senior center.

Subsequently, medical students also came to the center, under the direction of Dr. Rafael Lantigua, a geriatrician at Columbia. The questions to him were pointed: "What are you going to do for us? We're going to help you by giving medical students on-site training, but what will you provide for us? Every student requires more work on our part and we don't have a lot of workers." Dr. Lantigua calmly suggested, "Let's try it." As it happened, the medical students were field-testing the GERM (Geriatric Evaluation and Referral Model) instrument, which proved to be a very good tool and is now used in the Associates in Internal Medicine (AIM) practice at Columbia-Presbyterian. This became well-known and again increased the visibility of both the senior center and the AIM practice.

Moreover, the students became escorts for the clients of the center and helped them to get needed health care at Presbyterian Hospital. That is, medical students who were free on Friday afternoons decided to volunteer their time to serve as escorts of elderly clients.

The author gave visibility to this program by reporting on it at an annual meeting of the New York State Association of Gerontological Educators (SAGE). He had known nothing about this organization because his affiliates did not intersect with such groups. Rather, they tended to focus on on-line work and crises. It was clear that they needed to learn to work with other professional groups in the field, however. The presentation was a report on an interdisciplinary team, probably one of the first such teams developed, that included an occupational therapist, a nurse, an internist and a psychiatrist. The senior center did not have to pay for either the team or travel to the SAGE meeting because all expenses were picked up by Columbia University as teaching and training costs. In addition to on-site training, the hospital gained patients. Even though the senior center was near the hospital, its members were using it infrequently for several reasons: sometimes they became disoriented trying to find it; other times, they felt the hospital treated them badly. Elderly people need one-on-one care and having medical students at the center enabled its provision on-site. Furthermore, physicians were reimbursed for the care they provided at the senior center. Thus it worked out advantageously for all and the interdisciplinary team model practiced there became well-known.

FUNDING

Another coalition, called Alter Budget, which includes an aging section, was formed to develop an alternative to the New York City Mayor's budget. This coalition's position is that human services are just as important as police, fire and emergency services. The aging lobby joined this coalition only lately; the Mental Health Council, the Food and Hunger Council and the Council for the Homeless were members from the outset.

Because of pressure from the Alter Budget Coalition, money was added to New York City's budget to supplement the EISEP funding that had come down from New York State (see John Wren in this volume). EISEP guidelines had created difficulties: funds had not been allocated for emergency services or for people who needed fewer than four hours of case assistance weekly. Alter Budget caused $2 million to be added to the city budget to address these problems.

The Alter Budget Coalition is also working on the issue of home care. New York City's Home Care Council set up a home attendant program that lacks adequate supervision, case management or training, while still spending $700 million annually. It would seem, however, that little planning is occurring. Even though it was known 20 years ago that New York City would have a large aging population by the year 2000, day-to-day crises preclude any thoughtful, rational planning.

The Alter Budget Coalition meets bi-monthly with both the New York City Department for the Aging (DFTA) and the Human Resources Administration (HRA). A fact that has emerged from these meetings is that while there are social day care programs in New York City, DFTA will not recognize this modality, because it does not want to open up a new entitlement. Again, financial considerations determine everything. However, the coalition persuaded DFTA to set up a Social Day Care Task Force; this will, in all likelihood, lead to funding of these programs soon.

The real benefit of conferences such as this one is that participants can raise and discuss important issues. Such exchanges of ideas are extremely helpful in planning lobbying strategies to meet the needs of the elderly.

PLANNING

The issue of planning, or rather the lack of it due to the crisis-driven mentality in New York City, was alluded to earlier. A report by the Commission on the Year 2000, written for New York City, contained only three paragraphs on aging in this, the nation's largest city. Thus, there is no blueprint for what will happen to the aged in the year 2000. The Council of Senior Centers and Services of New York City has met with DFTA to discuss priorities for this milestone year.

Many problems concerning EISEP (which involved a major restructuring of programs in New York City to expand in-home services), DRGs, RUGs and DRUGs (Day Care Resource Utilization Groups) must be considered. The Council of Senior Centers and Services of New York City has turned to Columbia University researchers (e.g., Lois Grau) to interpret evaluations of these programs and their implications for planning.

Another planning activity that involved the author with researchers was Ft. Washington Houses. The Washington Heights-Inwood Council on the Aging, concerned about providing enriched housing for the elderly in the Washington Heights community, saw the potential in the former Delafield Hospital, which had become an eyesore since its closure. The Council on Aging, Community Board 12, elected officials, the New York City Health Department, Presbyterian Hospital and the New York City Housing Authority worked together and reached agreement to convert that building into purpose-built housing for the elderly. (See David Wilder's presentation, pp. 49-51, for a complete discussion of Ft. Washington Houses.) The pressure brought to bear on Presbyterian Hospital provides a rich lesson in how community groups can organize to become powerful, effective forces. The project took some eight years, from initial planning to successful completion; resistance from the hospital was strong.

The Washington Heights-Inwood Council on Aging was able, however, to convince Presbyterian Hospital to establish five primary-care group practices in the area, to compensate for the steady loss of private practitioners in the Washington Heights community (mostly due to retirement without replacement). One of these new group practices, the Ambulatory Care Network Corporation (based at Ft. Washington Houses) proved to be a model of primary geriatric medical care: it is well-staffed, it treats patients in a very individualized way and it provides follow-up care. All health professionals concerned with medical care of the elderly should visit this exemplary program.

This paper has offered numerous illustrations of how coalitions, be they community-based or city- or state-wide, can address successfully problems related to advocacy, visibility, funding and planning. Coalitions are a particularly effective strategy in these areas: individual agencies cannot possible wield the influence necessary to overcome bureaucratic obstacles. New York City has borough-wide Councils on Aging in each borough: the Bronx and Brooklyn councils are particularly strong, while Manhattan's has just been formed. The extent to which elected officials (borough presidents and others) work to procure funding for these councils is one reliable measure of their effectiveness: the Brooklyn and Queens councils have been very successful, whereas the Washington Heights-Inwood Council on Aging, with an annual budget of only $1,800 and a part-time secretary, managed to develop Alzheimer's respite, meals-on-wheels and large-scale transportation programs, by raising the requisite funds privately. This non-dependence on public monies has enabled the council to speak openly and critically of public policies and to represent people who are unable to make their own case.

One problem coalition-building per se cannot solve is the labor shortage: there is a desperate need for home attendants and case managers. Low salaries and lack of pensions for some workers (e.g., senior center directors) hardly attract the talent needed to develop and maintain vital service programs.

In summary, coalition-building is a struggle: great perseverance is needed just to keep going. Victories are generally modest: getting a health department to accept and support concepts such as socialization and social day care is perceived as a major accomplishment. But there is no other way to achieve the gains necessary to ensure that all elderly persons in the community are well-served.

Special Populations

Douglas Holmes, PhD

The term "special populations" refers generally to the minority elderly in this country; research has shown that, compared with all other elderly, they are particularly frail and vulnerable people. They are apt to be less healthy and their life expectancy is less than that of other elderly. As a rule, they are also less well-connected to community services. One would expect, therefore, that service agencies (such as Area Agencies on Aging) would make extra efforts to locate and serve these minority elderly, and that as a result, AAAs and other agencies would be serving them disproportionately. In fact, research on programs funded by AAAs indicates that up to 28% of these agencies served *less* than a proportionate share of minority elderly. That is, the proportion of minority elderly being served was less than their proportion in the total elderly population in the service areas of more than a quarter of the AAAs surveyed.

This research suggests that services are not being targeted adequately to minority elderly. Other research corroborates this, but the message has not been communicated loudly enough. Planners and providers alike persist in believing that special efforts are indeed being made to reach minority elderly and therefore special results are being effected and that the status quo is thus satisfactory. This is not the case.

It is helpful to consider obstacles to minority participation in community-based programs. Among the better-known are lack of knowledge on the part of minority elderly, language barriers, cultural differences and discrimination. Geographical dispersion is another obstacle, but it is less likely to be recognized, since the phenomenon occurs among only certain minority populations. For example, Japanese elderly tend to be dispersed geographically throughout the community. One does not find high-density Japanese areas analogous to the quite-common high density Chinese areas. This creates special problems in the planning and implementation of programs and, consequently, special barriers to the delivery of services to these elderly.

Having established that services to the minority are woefully inadequate, or at least proportionally inadequate, what, then, are service models? In global terms, there are two service models: the integrated service model and the segregated service model. The integrated model is well-understood and widely supported, for it sounds good, apart from being a viable model for service delivery. In contrast, segregated doesn't sound good, for historical reasons and because of the emotional responses the term engenders, particularly when applied to minority groups. In fact, there is a very definite need to be aware of and to use a segregated service model, particularly in response to the needs of geographically dispersed populations (e.g., Japanese elderly) and those that are high-density (e.g., Hispanic populations and high-density Asian-American populations)—all require a service-segregated model. Although this would seem to be obvious, there is often such a value attached to integration that program planners try to impose an integrated model, even in situations which clearly don't support it.

Within the integrated model there are a few observations that should be made. The first observation addresses creation of what has been termed an "ethnic ramp" into the program—a term coined long ago when nutrition programs were trying to attract people from all sources by distributing flyers to churches, paying occasional visits to senior centers or other similar efforts. These approaches are quite inadequate for minority populations. It is absolutely essential that an ethnic ramp be created wherein personal contact is made with minority group members in a target area. This may consist of having staff people who are themselves minority people visit locations from which a program is trying to recruit people and having them establish a personal contact with people in that location, thereby bringing them into the program. This constitutes an effective ethnic ramp. The term is very apt, because it suggests a sequence of attraction, recruitment, enrollment, involvement and maintenance of minority group people in ongoing programs.

The second observation concerns the unrealistic and ineffective notion of the "color-blind" approach. This is reflected in the frequently heard claim of, "Oh, we don't notice whether a person is black or white or whatever—it doesn't make a difference to us. We're color blind. We just have programs for people." This shows a good egalitarian/libertarian instinct but is not conducive to recognizing and addressing the very special needs of different populations and subpopulations. Thus it is absolutely necessary to get away from the color-blind orientation and to recognize that within any particular minority constituency there are also vast differences among subgroups. For this reason, a good segregated model in an agency of any size at all requires the formation of a task force, such as a unit on the board of directors—a viable working body that includes members of the minority group but which can reflect a number of different views. Many agencies attempt to manage by designating *a* minority person to be responsible for addressing the needs of *the* minority in their area. However, *the* minority may, in fact, be a number of subminorities or subgroups among the minorities and that one poor staff person is expected not only to accommodate the needs and cultural differences of all these people but to exercise sufficient clout to create and implement a program as well. It is essential in every agency that a group (e.g., a task force) be charged with the tasks of identifying the target group; identifying subgroups among that target group; identifying the needs of each of these groups, as different as they may be; and assuming responsibility for developing specific policies in response to each of these identified needs. Again, specificity of recognition and planning are absolutely fundamental to the creation of any viable, successful program for minority elderly. Experience has shown that program planners and providers too often overlook or minimize these critical elements.

The third observation is the need to collect good data concerning the participation of minorities. One responsibility of service planners is to set goals and objectives, and there is no substitute for the collection of good, hard, objective data to determine whether these objectives are being met. Data must be collected during the implementation and operation of service programs, not only to assess goal achievement, but to enable the making of necessary program adjustments to keep things on track.

The last observation concerns training, for which there are a number of good programs. New York State, for example, with support from the Administration on Aging, has a minority internship program in which students who are minority group members are attached to Area Agencies on Aging and deal with services for minorities. It is, therefore, a training and service program and offers an incredible opportunity to train indigenous personnel. Invariably, service agencies are excellent workshops, or laboratories, in which students can learn first-hand the realities of providing services to all elderly people. Experience with special needs of minority populations is a critical element in the learning experience.

Filling the Housing and Service Gap

David Wilder, PhD

From the perspective of housing and the elderly, two major issues are highly interconnected. One is the issue of affordability of housing, and the other is the issue of providing a variety of services to the people who increasingly need them, as they become older and more frail and dependent. Specialists concerned with housing needs of the elderly within the context of long term care must, of course, address both these issues. And they both must be seen against the peculiar demographics and housing situations of the elderly in this country. Most people don't realize that the majority of elderly people in this country now live in the suburbs. Indeed, the majority of all people in this country now live in the suburbs. And yet the suburbs are primarily a post-World War II phenomenon. About three-fourths of people over the age of 65 own their own homes. About one-third live alone, and this increases significantly as they become older. Thus, substantial numbers of the elderly are becoming increasingly frail and are frequently living alone and in need of services. Providing programs that respond to all these needs is extremely difficult. The long term care challenge becomes how to alter existing environments to accommodate the disabled; how to provide services within the community; and how to get the elderly who are in need of these services into such environments where this can be done economically and without displacing already existing support systems. It may not be possible for many of these elderly to stay in their own homes, but there have to be more alternatives to traditional institutional settings.

Although most elderly people live in suburban communities, urban environments often offer the best opportunities to take existing space in buildings no longer in use, such as factories and schools, and to convert it into purposefully-designed housing that can ac-

49

commodate frail, dependent elderly people. A very innovative example of such a conversion exists in Manhattan's Washington Heights. Delafield Hospital, a part of Columbia-Presbyterian Medical Center, was closed in the 1970s; vandals promptly reduced it to a locus of crime and an eyesore. There have been extensive ethnic and economic changes in the neighborhood around the Medical Center. The poverty level has been increasing steadily. There has also been an influx of Spanish-speaking and elderly people in the neighborhood.

Recognizing the potential of the abandoned hospital for conversion to purpose-built housing for the elderly, the community forged a coalition to rescue it. This coalition included representatives of Fort Washington Houses Services for the Elderly, Inc. (a newly-formed organization), Columbia-Presbyterian Medical Center, the Washington Heights-Inwood Council on Aging, the New York City Department for the Aging, the New York City Housing Authority and all politicians whose districts include Washington Heights. Not only was Delafield Hospital spared demolition, but it was converted into a model of planned housing for the elderly, thanks to a determined community coalition.

Today, Fort Washington Houses comprises three, interrelated parts: 225 apartments, which are all wheelchair-accessible and equipped with handrails and call buttons, comprising the actual houses; a senior center for residents of the houses, as well as other community elderly (Fort Washington Services for the Elderly, Inc.); and the Ambulatory Care Network Corporation, a fully-staffed clinic which operates out of Presbyterian Hospital. Services to residents of Fort Washington Houses include home attendants, supplied by CASA (some twenty-five residents have them); transportation, provided by nearby ARC-Ft. Washington Senior Center; a resident advisor, who is provided by New York City Housing Authority and who is available around the clock; and weekend meals-on-wheels, which is supplied by Isabella Geriatric Center and needed only on weekends, because during the week all residents, no matter how frail or without home attendants, manage to get to the Senior Center nutrition site downstairs.

Fort Washington Services to the Elderly, Inc., the on-premises senior center/nutrition site, occupies some 25,000 square feet indoors, plus a protected outdoors area. Over the years, it has evolved into a comprehensive senior center. Of its 900 members, 200 are residents of the houses. Their demographics generally reflect those of the elderly in the Washington Heights neighborhood: 71% are at or below the poverty line; 60% live alone; 62% are Hispanic; 59% speak no English; 17% are black; 15% are white.

The old Delafield Hospital, reborn and thriving as a model of how the housing and service gap can be filled, is now a showplace, an exemplary place to see an incredible variety of organizations working together, reaching out into the community, providing ambulatory and primary care, and providing emergency services for residents of the houses. The Senior Center even operates a Lombardi Bill ("Nursing Home without Walls") home health care program for elderly in the neighboring community—truly the art of the possible. Every community with a vacant building—hospital, school, factory—could, with requisite determination and effort, replicate the Fort Washington Houses success story.

PART II:
THE ROLE OF COLLEGES AND UNIVERSITIES IN TRAINING PERSONNEL TO DEVELOP COMMUNITY-BASED LONG TERM CARE SERVICES

Introduction to Part II

As was indicated earlier, one of the chief concerns that prompted the conference on which this book is based was how to teach graduate students in the Division of Geriatrics and Gerontology, Columbia University School of Public Health, about community-based long term care for the elderly. While there are well-developed curricula in gerontology and, to some extent, in long term care, there is very little available on community-based long term care because this field is in its infancy. There is a high probability, however, that new graduates of programs such as that in the Division of Geriatrics and Gerontology will be asked to work in, administer, plan for and develop community-based long term care services and programs for the elderly. Undoubtedly, that is the wave of the future.

Clearly, if the Division is to teach students about community-based long term care services, it must familiarize them with such services. But more than that, it must select from the maze of ser-

53

vices and agencies those that appear to be doing an exemplary job and are willing to accept Division students for practica, site visits and internships. In addition, administrators and others are asked routinely to lecture to Division students about the day-to-day operations of their agencies and programs, as well as to be open and honest about problems encountered, unmet needs of the agencies and the elderly in general and policy issues that might affect their work. These matters were addressed, to some extent, in the previous section of this book.

Part II describes the training experiences developed for students in the Division's Master of Public Health (MPH) program with a specialization in long term care administration as well as for students in related programs. All of the chapters here address training issues with a focus on working with the community-based elderly. These training approaches have evolved over time and are still evolving, especially because the community-based long term care field is still evolving and changing.

The first chapter, by Ruth Bennett and Susana Frisch, is on "The Master of Public Health (MPH) Program in Long Term Care Administration at the Columbia University School of Public Health." This program was developed within the Division of Geriatrics and Gerontology under a 17-month grant from the Administration on Aging (AoA). A major goal of this program from the outset was to familiarize students with community-based long term care services for the elderly.

Eloise Killeffer describes in the second chapter "The Practicum Experience," which is required of all candidates for the MPH degree within the Program in Long Term Care Administration. The practicum experience is required because many students have not encountered elderly persons except, perhaps, for family members. It is simply unwise to graduate persons who have not tried to work with elderly people. Course work is not an adequate substitute for direct experience with the elderly.

Shura Saul describes the relationship between learning in the field and academic training in her chapter on "The Relationship Between Field Placement Agencies and the University." She elaborates on the basic components of the field experience: the student, the university and the agency within which the field experience occurs.

K. Della Ferguson, in her chapter "Training for Community Programs," describes a program, based at Utica College of Syracuse University, called PACE (Planning, Advocacy and Coordination for the Elderly), which trains students to work with caregivers, a vital link in the community-based service chain.

Lynn Tepper, in her chapter on "Outpatient Programs from the Training Point of View," describes her efforts to sensitize students in the School of Dental and Oral Surgery to the needs of elderly patients served at the Columbia-Presbyterian Medical Center: "Geriatric Dentistry Training at Columbia University." Lucien Cote, in his presentation "Geriatric Medical Training at Columbia University," discusses analogous efforts in the College of Physicians & Surgeons.

In the last chapter, John Toner provides a complete training module on the "Long Term Care Service Continuum Model" as it is taught in his course "Overview of Long Term Care" in the Division of Geriatrics and Gerontology. This module is divided into six sessions, each of which contains content to be taught as well as issues to be emphasized and tips on how to do so. Readings relevant to each session are listed at the end of the chapter. His overview course is a required introductory course for all Division students. Annual course evaluations have shown the course to be popular and its content a revelation for many students, for whom long term care is synonymous with nursing home care. These students quickly learn that the term means much more and they generally are very enthusiastic about community-based alternatives. Unfortunately, their enthusiasm is often dampened by discussions of the patchwork nature of long term care service delivery. However, many have good ideas that may be realized one day if they continue to work in this field.

The MPH Program in Long Term Care Administration at the Columbia University School of Public Health

Ruth Bennett, PhD
Susana Frisch, MA

The Columbia University School of Public Health, through the Division of Geriatrics and Gerontology, offers a program with a major emphasis on the area of Long Term Care Administration. The program's goal is to train administrators, policy analysts, planners and researchers in institutional and community-based long term care. The student population of the School of Public Health includes health and human services professionals, such as nurses, physicians, social workers, occupational therapists and dentists; as well as administrators and workers currently employed in health care and social service facilities.

RATIONALE

Long term care is defined as the provision of one or more services on a sustained basis to enable individuals whose functional capacities are chronically impaired to be maintained at their maximum levels of health and well-being. A key focus of this program is to train gerontological professionals to identify those for whom long term care is appropriate, and to determine the nature of the services and the qualities of the environments that would maximize their well-being.

There is a need to provide a core of professional personnel aspiring to careers in long term care administration with the expertise and skills to address the complex issues in the field. The policy, financing, regulatory and programming issues in the field of long term care require intensive study by those entering the field of long term care administration. The ever-expanding knowledge areas of geriatrics and gerontology, combined with basic management skills, must be mastered by those responsible for day-to-day operations of long term care organizations. However, in order to go beyond day-to-day management crises and to be able to plan or evaluate, it is necessary to have public health skills that deal with populations and communities. Specifically, this involves the understanding of disease and social factors influencing the health of the elderly community; demography; and evaluation.

PROGRAM DESIGN

This program is designed to upgrade and expand the skills of students interested in long term care by adding to core public health training in biostatistics; epidemiology; environmental sciences; health care organization and social sciences; gerontological skills courses; courses in management, organizational theory, financing and economics; long term care policy; regulation; and programming. In addition, each student devotes four months full-time to a practicum with a preceptor who is an administrator or other managerial staff person in such organizations as area agencies on aging, community-based long term service agencies or long term care institutions.

The program is unique when compared to other programs because its primary emphasis is on having professionals trained in health fields address programs for the elderly as well as problems of populations and communities. It offers the quantitative tools necessary to identify problems, find interventions and evaluate the effects of those interventions to students who already have some health professional skills. Programs based primarily in management or public administration do not provide these skills or perspectives. At the same time, the School of Public Health provides high-quality instruction in management skills and strategy formulation, thus making possible the development of highly-competent managers and executives who take both a short- and long-term view of problems in long term care administration.

THE CURRICULUM

To receive the MPH degree, a student must complete 45 credits of academic study, a four-month practicum and a master's essay. The program can be pursued on a full-time or part-time basis. A full-time student can expect to earn the degree within two years (including two summers), depending upon the type of practicum selected.

Suggested Program Outline:
A. Core Public Health Courses (required)　　　　15 credits

  Medical Background (required of students without medical knowledge)
  Introduction to Biostatistics *or*
  Introduction to Biostatistical Methods
  Environmental Sciences
  Principles of Epidemiology
  Issues and Approaches in Health Administration
  Introduction to Sociomedical Sciences (*or* a substitute course approved by the Division of Sociomedical Sciences)
  Note: Waiver examinations are given at the beginning of each semester for the core courses (except Biostatistics, which gives a placement exam). Waiving out of any core course frees up 3 credits for use elsewhere in the curriculum.

B. Concentration Courses　　　　21 credits
　　　　　　　　　　　　　　(out of those listed)

  Overview of Geriatrics and Gerontology
  Overview of Long Term Care
  Assessment of Intellectual, Emotional and Physical Change in the Older Adult
  Interdisciplinary Collaboration in Long-Term Care: A Seminar and Practicum
  Long-Term Care Policy
  Regulation and Financing of Long-Term Care
  Long-Term Care Management and Administration

Long-Term Care Programming and Planning
Processes of Aging
Longevity
Mental Health of the Aged
Caregiving and Related Transitions in Midlife and Older
    Women

C. Selected Elective Courses   9 credits
    (taught in other divisions)

Organization Theory and Health Services
Health Care Financial Management
Political Economy of Health Care
Organizational and Community Linkages
Ethics as Applied to Health Care Administration
Issues and Approaches in Health Administration
Strategic Planning in Health Care Institutions
Preventive Medicine and Public Health
Women and Health
Social Aspects of Physical Disability and Rehabilitation
Social and Psychological Consequences of Institutional
    and Community Care
Tutorials (Division of Geriatrics & Gerontology)

D. Four-Month Practicum   0 credits

E. Master's Essay   0 credits

Admission Requirements

Applicants must have a bachelor's degree from a recognized college or university and must submit scores from the Graduate Record Examination or its equivalent. Professional experience in the fields of geriatrics or gerontology is highly desirable.

PROGRAM RESOURCES

The Columbia University School of Public Health is one of 24 accredited schools of public health in the United States. It has a large and distinguished interdisciplinary faculty and is dedicated to education, research and service involving the health of communities and populations. The school is currently organized into eight academic divisions providing both new knowledge and education in the skills and content needed to address problems of public health importance in this country and abroad. The school collaborates with eight other schools in the University in sponsoring joint programs of instruction: the Graduate School of Business; the Graduate School of Architecture; the School of Dental and Oral Surgery; the College of Physicians and Surgeons; the School of Social Work; the School of Nursing; the Programs in Occupational Therapy; and The Graduate Program in Public Policy and Administration. In addition, it collaborates formally with the Graduate Faculty of Arts and Sciences to offer the PhD degree in selected public health disciplines.

The Center for Geriatrics, Gerontology and Long Term Care, established in 1980, provides a working environment for a number of researchers, teachers and clinicians who have been involved in the field of aging for the greater part of their professional careers. The Center is supported by the Faculty of Medicine of Columbia University and the New York State Office of Mental Health. It is part of a large network of academic and service programs and has initiated collaborative ventures that have led to major developments in geriatric programs in the Schools of Medicine, Public Health and Dentistry; the Department of Psychiatry and the New York State Psychiatric Institute; the Programs in Occupational and Physical Therapy; the Presbyterian Hospital; and local community service agencies.

The Program Faculty

Division courses are taught by a multidisciplinary faculty and are enriched by the participation of guest University faculty lecturers and community leaders with recognized expertise in the field of aging and long term care.

Barry J. Gurland, MD, Head, Division of Geriatrics and Gerontology; Director, Center for Geriatrics and Gerontology; and John E. Borne Professor of Clinical Psychiatry, Faculty of Medicine
Ruth G. Bennett, PhD, Director of Graduate Studies, Division of Geriatrics and Gerontology; Deputy Director, Center for Geriat-

rics and Gerontology; Professor of Clinical Public Health (in the Center for Geriatrics and Gerontology in Psychiatry)

John A. Toner, EdD, Research Scientist, Center for Geriatrics and Gerontology; Assistant Professor of Clinical Public Health

Abraham Monk, PhD, Professor of Social Work; Brookdale Professor of Gerontology, Columbia University School of Social Work

Patricia A. Miller, MEd, OTR, Assistant Professor of Clinical Occupational Therapy, Columbia University Programs in Occupational Therapy

Lynn Tepper, EdD, Assistant Professor of Clinical Dentistry, Columbia University School of Dental and Oral Surgery

Shura Saul, EdD, ACSW, Lecturer

Eloise H. P. Killeffer, EdM, Senior Research Scientist, Center for Geriatrics and Gerontology; Practicum Coordinator and Administrator, Division of Geriatrics and Gerontology

Practicum Sites

Practicum sites include all settings where long-term care of the elderly is a primary concern, from community-based direct service agencies to institutional settings to social and health planning agencies to the legislative arena. To the maximum extent possible, each student is placed in a setting whose activities are most consonant with his/her professional goals and career interests. It is also possible for students already working in appropriate agencies to do their practica there, under certain specified constraints. It should also be noted that there are no geographical limitations on the practicum, so it is not compulsory to do it in New York City proper.

Examples of possible practicum sites include the following (most are located within the five boroughs of New York City):

— Bronx Field Office on Aging (a branch of the New York City Department for the Aging, which is itself an Area Agency on Aging)

— Riverdale Senior Services, Inc. (a case-managed coordinated service delivery agency in the West Bronx)

— ARC-Ft. Washington Senior Center (a multi-purpose senior center)

— Volunteer Services for the Elderly of Yorkville, Inc.

—ICD Day Care Program for Alzheimer's Patients
—Kingsbridge Heights Lombardi Bill Home Care Program
—Kingsbridge Heights Geriatric Center
—Village Nursing Home
—Westchester County Office for the Aging
—New York Service Program for Older People, Inc. (SPOP)
—Morningside House Nursing Home Corporation, Inc.

The practicum is described in full in the next chapter.

The Practicum Experience

Eloise H. P. Killeffer, EdM

The MPH in Long Term Care Administration degree program, offered by the Division of Geriatrics and Gerontology, Columbia University School of Public Health, has been developed in recognition of the nation's increasing need for skilled health professionals who are well-grounded in all aspects of care of the elderly: core public health skills (biostatistics, epidemiology, environmental sciences, health care organization); administrative skills (management, organizational theory, financing, economics, long term care policy, regulation, programming, interdisciplinary collaboration); and gerontological skills (assessment, physical/mental/social aspects of aging).

The practicum is intended to serve an integrative and connective function, enabling the student to apply in a real-life situation the extensive classroom learning he/she has acquired. It is also intended to serve as the basis for the required master's essay, in which the student discusses his/her practicum project within the larger context of gerontological theory and practice.

The administrative philosophies, knowledge and skills deemed essential to good administrative practice in today's complex arena of long term care have been incorporated into all required courses in the program as appropriate and should receive equal emphasis in the practicum, which is, after all, an integral part of the curriculum. While the knowledge that is imparted in the classroom and the limited experience gained in a four-month practicum cannot produce "instant administrators," they should, together, give students valid criteria by which to judge and define good administrative practices by themselves and others.

It is therefore essential that all participants in the practicum—student, faculty advisor, preceptor, agency—understand and support the practicum experience. Its success requires a substantial investment of time, cooperation and teamwork, but the potential dividends — well-trained and motivated administrators prepared to assume responsible, contributive roles in the long term care system — are too great to permit compromise.

DESCRIPTION OF THE PRACTICUM
IN LONG TERM CARE ADMINISTRATION

The practicum is required of students working for the MPH in Long Term Care Administration (LCTA) degree. The faculty believe that every MPH candidate in this Division, even established professionals, will derive great benefit from the practicum experience. Consequently, the requirement is waived only under the most unusual circumstances. Because of the program's strong emphasis on extra-institutional administration (e.g., programs and agencies other than long term care facilities), the Division of Geriatrics and Gerontology has developed new linkages (and strengthened existing ties) with an array of national, state and local agencies involved with all aspects of long term care: direct service provision; policy development and analysis; policy implementation; research; and teaching/education. Students can thus select from a great variety of possible practicum sites, thereby maximizing the potential for compatibility with career interests.

Although the LTCA practicum is generally thought of as a four-month, full-time experience, students whose needs dictate may modify that schedule, subject to approval by the practicum agency, the Practicum Coordinator and the student's academic advisor. Thus it may be more practical to define the practicum in terms of hours: approximately 600, occurring within an agreed-upon number of months.

Because of this program's emphasis on extra-institutional administration, one aspect of long term care administration is not addressed by the practicum as currently structured: nursing home administration. That is, the four-month practicum does not meet requirements of either New York State (nine months) or New Jersey (six months) for pre-licensure on-site experience. Students who wish to sit for nursing home administrator licensure examinations will find the 45 credits of course work highly relevant to the licensure requirements. However, special arrangements will have to be made among the School of Public Health, the particular state licensing agency and a long term care facility approved by that state to provide administrative residencies, in order to enable a student to obtain the experience required for nursing home licensure.

The practicum is undertaken (with limited exceptions) after the student has completed the 45 credits of course work required for the MPH in Long Term Care Administration degree. There is no stipulation of when in the calendar year the practicum must begin, unless the particular agency chosen has preferences or restrictions. Many students find summer (May-August or June-September) a convenient time for the practicum.

Students who enter the program as established professionals already employed in an appropriate setting may want to do their practicum at their place of employment, although specific restrictions are attached to such an arrangement.

The practicum is a learning experience in the real world of the long term care system. Its value to the student of gerontological administration derives from its experiential nature: i.e., there are whole areas of learning through working and observing that cannot be taught anywhere but in the field. Thus the practicum is more than "enhancement of classroom learning" or "application of theory to practice." Rather, it is that part of the total curriculum wherein the student can combine the learning of classroom and literature with that which is actively inherent in practice. Further, it enables the student to experience what has been conceptualized in lecture, literature review and classroom interaction and to conceptualize the learning of real-life situations. Through these connections, the student may develop an integrated, in-depth approach to the philosophy, the theory, the practice and the ongoing discovery and learning in the practice of long term care administration.

It is critical that this concept of the practicum is understood and accepted by the agency in which the student is placed, for a successful practicum requires a mutual investment by student, faculty and agency in the teaching/learning potential of the setting as well as in the total experience.

THE ADMINISTRATOR IN LONG TERM CARE

The faculty of the Division of Geriatrics and Gerontology has identified particular administrative philosophies, knowledge and skills as being essential to good administrative practice in the increasingly complex system of long term care. These management tools are basic and fundamental, and are not affected by changing fashions in regulation and reimbursement. Further, they are useful and usable across the spectrum of long term care settings, from senior centers to skilled nursing facilities. It is essential that all participants in the practicum — student, faculty, agency administrator, preceptor — have a common and complete understanding of the objectives of this gerontological administration curriculum, including the practicum. (*Note: These elements are given in outline form here; they are discussed in full in the Manual for the Practicum, available from the author of this article.*)

1. Clarity of administrative philosophy: Purposes and goals of long term care administration
2. Historical perspective: Understanding social policy and legislation as they affect elderly people, their families and long term care
3. Areas of knowledge:
   a. Understanding aging as part of a lifespan development process
   b. Understanding aging in the context of today's attitudes and lifestyles
   c. The epidemiology of the social conditions of aging in the 1980s
   d. The impact of contemporary social circumstances on the life and inner self of the older person
   e. The changing needs of people in the "third trimester" of life (which may encompass three decades or more): e.g., the need for equilibrium in the face of altered balance between independence and dependency and the roles of change and loss and their stressful impact on the aging person
   f. Unique aspects of normal identity crises (inherent in all de-

velopmental stages) during the aging process (a less-well understood stage)

g. Interaction among physical, psychological, intellectual and emotional dimensions of self; the impact of changes within each upon each other and upon the whole person

h. Coping with changes, both planned and unplanned

i. Coping with losses

j. Concepts of death and dying (one's own death and the deaths of significant others)

k. Understanding the specific impact of health loss on the aging individual and on the family

l. The nature of chronic illness and disability; their impact on individual and family life and on relationships; the consequent needs of individual and family for understanding, services and care

m. Health promotion and illness prevention

n. Etiology of mental illnesses that may develop during the aging process; understanding possible causes; reversibility and treatment possibilities; specific types and qualities of mental illnesses (particularly depression, but covering the range of emotional states and unusual behaviors)

o. Consumer education, especially in health promotion and illness prevention; use of medications; and need for continuity of lifestyle, of emotional, creative and intellectual experiences and of appropriate socialization

p. Understanding the patient/client and family in the long term care system; understanding the effect on the patient during and after entry into the long term care system (whether in the community or in an institution, the patient/client responds to changed needs, roles and status that accompany this entry)

q. Knowledge and understanding of family relationships, to gain perspective on the dynamics of the three- and four-generation family as well as insight into specific, individual family situations

r. Understanding the effects of ethnicity, religion, ethics, individual and family philosophy and values, class and culture-related value systems on the individual's behavior and expectations of and attitudes toward society, life and death

s. General understanding of the range of treatment modalities and their applicability and potential usefulness to the patient/client and family in long term care

t. Understanding of community resources and how to use them on behalf of patients/clients and family in long term care

u. Understanding of the long term care system's contribution to the community

v. Awareness of current social policy and legislation and how they affect long term care

w. Understanding how to relate to the social policy system and how to influence necessary change

THE PRACTICUM FOR ADMINISTRATION IN LONG TERM CARE

Many agencies have long-standing relationships with college or university programs that place students of more conventional disciplines (e.g., social work, nursing, occupational therapy, physical therapy, even medicine and dentistry). Most such placements are very structured, with specification of required activities, scrupulous accounting of time, extensive record-keeping and even assigned sites.

The practicum required of students in the MPH program in long term care administration is markedly different in many respects. Within certain limitations, it is a much more flexible (e.g., much less structured) experience. Students select agencies whose activities are consonant with their own career interests and goals. When the student-agency match has been arranged, the student and his/her preceptor, in consultation with the Division's Practicum Coordinator and the student's academic advisor, identify the focus of the practicum experience, including a specific project the student will work on.

Once the student has become oriented to the agency, its activities and its staff, it is expected that he/she will assume the confidence to work as independently as the circumstances permit. Many students come into the program with formal professional training (e.g., nursing or social work) and all come to the practicum with all (or most) of 45 credits of the MPH course work completed. Thus they are mature, knowledgeable and skilled, and ready to be integrated into the agencies' normal operations.

The practicum may be seen as an apprenticeship, wherein the student is "apprenticed" to the designated mentor, who will not only teach and guide the student, but will serve as a good role model as well. Although there is much flexibility in the nature and structure of each practicum, it is expected that certain criteria will be met.

The practicum should be designed individually to meet the general and specific learning needs of the student, and should take into account the student's experience, talents and background, as well as gaps in knowledge and experience. It should be built around the student's career goals but should not be narrow in focus.

If the student has had no prior experience with elderly persons, the practicum should provide opportunity for exposure and direct, first-hand experience with them at more than one point in the service continuum (e.g., well elderly in a prevention program as well as frail elderly in a service-intensive program). If the student has had some experience with elderly persons, the practicum should offer additional dimensions (e.g., if the student's experience has been in institutional settings, the practicum should somehow touch on community settings). Further, if the student has not had prior experience with families, effort should be directed toward including some aspect of this.

Direct contact with the elderly is essential, regardless of the nature of the practicum (research as well as service-oriented). A research project should not remove the student from contact with the elderly as well as with agencies (and their staffs) who serve them.

The practicum should involve the student in a learning-and-doing experience, the outcomes of which benefit the student, the agency/ program and the clients being served. The student should be giving as well as receiving in the practicum.

The practicum should be designed to include opportunities to practice in the long term care system and to study and interpret the practice experience with the assistance of, and in consultation with, supervisory and teaching expertise in both class and field. It may be seen as a laboratory experience in these respects: (1) practice exercises (experiences, including observations) and work assignments are developed in individually appropriate and diversified ways; (2) approaches to tasks are studied, planned and tested; (3) plans are implemented; (4) suitable records are maintained; (5) evaluative methods are developed; (6) a range of opportunities is employed consistently to study, evaluate, learn, correct and create; (7) insights are achieved and conclusions are drawn; and (8) learning is related to theoretical concepts and constructs.

The practicum should afford a variety of learning opportunities and experiences, with particular emphasis on interdisciplinary collaboration and interchange. Sufficient time should be allowed to analyze all practicum experiences in depth and such analysis should employ a variety of methods (e.g., conferences, documentation, group seminars and supervision). There must be opportunities to experiment with methods of recording and evaluation and with approaches to practice. Finally, the practicum must afford the student a chance to contribute constructively and usefully to the host agency, in return for the time, support and other resources invested in the student.

A complete Practicum Manual is available from the author of this article.

The Relationship Between Field Placement Agencies and the University

Shura Saul, EdD, ACSW

There is a substantial amount of significant learning by students placed in field agencies. This learning is indigenous to the field experience, is both theoretical and practical in nature and coincides with, but also differs from, classroom material. It is not, as some professors may think, adjunctive to classroom learning. Nor is it, as some field instructors seem to think, more important. Neither extreme is the case. There is nothing in the field to replace the disciplined and orderly presentation, conceptualization and gathering of knowledge and theory offered in the classroom. Nor is there anything to replace, or simulate, the real-life situations and accompanying learning in the world of work with people. In training for any role in the field of human services and long term health care, both learning opportunities must be viewed as complementary.

There are three basic components of the field experience, and each of these is complex in itself. First is the student: a person with individual learning needs, goals, experience and talent and a mixed constellation of personal past and present, all of which affect his/her needs and expectations in the practicum. Second is the university: a complex of requirements, expectations and relationships, all of which affect and direct the student. The agency must understand these two components, if the student's experience is to be fulfilling and satisfactory. The university is personalized through the presence of the faculty (or practicum) advisor on the field experience scene. Like all other human beings, faculty advisors have their individual styles, interpret university rules in various ways and relate to different students differently. Thus the faculty person must be understood by the other principals in this complex triumvirate. The third component is the agency itself, with its own goals, purposes

73

and commitments to clients, regulating agencies, and whatever other powers control its existence. In the case of field instruction, the agency is usually personalized by the field instructor or supervisor, who also has a unique style. Thus there are three individuals, from three different arenas, each with a complex agenda. The three agendas coincide in two areas: in the student's learning program and in the principals' mutual concern for excellence in long term care.

The model, used by the author for more than twenty years, attempts to emphasize all the positive contributions of each member of this triumvirate, to create a *troika*, as it were, in which each member offers leadership and input toward a desired goal. The goal, of course, is the successful completion of an individual learning program designed to capitalize on the student's strengths in an educational experience that offers new learning. There are many steps toward this goal.

AGENCY/SCHOOL RELATIONSHIP

The school usually locates the agency whose functions are relevant to the school program and the student's learning needs and which is organized and integrated so as to accommodate a non-staff member (i.e., the student) in the combined work-learning role. This relationship, critical to the student's development, is generally established through the administrator, whose investment in the teaching component of the agency is of primary importance. The other critical ongoing relationship in this picture exists between the faculty advisor and the field instructor, the details of which become clear as the process is described.

Agency Preparation

Preparation of the agency itself is a task whose importance must not be underestimated. Like any field which is to yield growth, it must be readied for the planting. This is the task for the field instructor or in more sophisticated settings "the coordinator of training." The entire agency, from administrator to all staff to clients and, where relevant, to families, must be aware of, and appreciate the presence and contribution of the student. The student's role is not always easy to define. Why is he/she there? The educational agent's reply is simple: the student is there to learn, and everyone in the agency, including clients, is part of the learning process. Learning is derived through experience, service and interpretation.

The Learning Process

The learning program itself must be individualized for each student and is determined by the three principals involved: student, field instructor, faculty advisor. Their decisions are based on the student's learning needs, an assessment of which is derived from an evaluation of his/her level of knowledge, skills, experience and individual learning goals. This assessment is made very early in the relationship and shapes the student's individual assignment within the agency.

The Assignment

The assignment itself derives from the needs of the agency and its clients, blended with the student's learning needs. It is here that the creativity of the field instructor is tested. What can the student give to the setting, while deriving the specific learning he/she requires? How does one fit the student into the *gestalt* of the agency and its services? Constant interpretation to the agency is necessary to ensure that the student's needs, and not the agency's, are primary. If the agency suggests a task that fits the student's needs, the field instructor, faculty advisor and student can work it out. But sometimes, an agency request for the student's assistance may be inappropriate in terms of the student's learning program; this must then be interpreted to the agency by the field instructor.

The Client

The client, who is often very needy and whose problems are the student's *raison d'etre* is also important in the agency. In the best situation, it is anticipated that the student will develop relationships with clients, for it is through these relationships and the insights they yield that much learning occurs. The client, however, is not concerned with student learning needs, but with his or her needs.

The client's relationship to the agency is predicated on the agency's meeting those needs. Consequently, client requests, even demands, of students may not be in keeping with the student's learning program. Again, such requests require scrutiny and professional assessment by both student and field instructor. The student must learn to discern how much acquiescence to client request is appropriate and what part is relevant to learning. Many things we do for clients are part of any human relationship — this too becomes part of the learning experience, especially when the interpretive process is applied.

Relationships Within the Agency

This additional complex of relationships within the agency (e.g., student, agency, client) must be understood by all parties including the school. Any negotiations among them become the primary responsibility of the field instructor and/or student coordinator. Matters here may sometimes become very sensitive and in the final analysis, the agency must leave the ultimate decision to the field instructor or student coordinator. Should matters become extremely difficult, the faculty advisor may become involved.

The Interpretive Learning Process

Experience without interpretation has limited value. People learn from their own insights. Experiences, relationships, mistakes, triumphs, critical events, even the tiniest — seemingly trivial — interactions form the basis for these insights. In the model offered here, it is suggested that the learning-teaching relationship between student and field instructor becomes the lens of a microscope, as it were, through which experiences are examined, analyzed and discussed. Hindsight being unerringly 20/20, this process can be very useful.

The field instructor, together with the student, develops tools through which experiential information may be processed. These may be logs, diaries or records of different types. There should be a regularly set time for student-instructor conferences, during which these records of experience are discussed and analyzed. The field instructor also employs other teaching materials, e.g., tapes, films and special readings.

Learning in the field involves exposure to material that is theoretical as well as practical. The field instructor should make available readings which can help the student in the specific learning situation. Very often incidents, problems and concerns that have not yet been dealt with in class arise in the field. The field instructor helps the student understand these in the most generic and profound way: that is, the basic concepts underlying practice approaches must be taught in the field as the need arises. Finally, fieldwork learning involves the process of connecting some of the theoretical class material with the real-life situations. Often, these are not recognized easily by the student. The field instructor has the responsibility of helping the student identify such situations and make the necessary corrections.

THE MULTI-FACETED ROLE
OF THE FIELD INSTRUCTOR

The role of field instructor is extraordinarily critical. The true teacher will find ways to make every experience contribute to the student's learning. The atmosphere in which the material is discussed must be non-judgmental, supportive and conducive to honest and sincere analysis.

Ongoing Evaluation

As the student progresses in understanding, new learning goals may be set and new tasks developed to enable those goals to be achieved. Evaluation, therefore, is ongoing and communication among agency, student and school remains open. If the student does not seem to be learning in reasonably satisfactory ways or at an acceptable rate, the field instructor, together with the student, examines the problem and restructures the learning plan. The school faculty advisor is involved in this process, at the request of the instructor or the student — preferably both. As a field instructor herself, the author has never turned to the faculty advisor without first involving the student. Three-way conferences are an excellent vehicle for correcting plans and expectations and for making changes. In this model, the involvement of the student is again a teaching device, for the student learns about open communication, self-evaluation and correction — all important skills in the human services.

This model has proven useful, because all involved are able to achieve desired goals. The student learns through doing, through being guided and through ongoing interpretation of the entire experience. The agency gains a dedicated newcomer, one who enhances service through the acceptance of a work assignment needed by the agency. The client gains from the student's contribution to the agency, either directly or indirectly. Not so incidentally, it is a good idea to build in opportunities for the student to report to others in the agency; this adds a dimension of staff development, another plus for the agency. Sometimes a student is able to make some suggestions to enhance agency functioning or service. When the agency environment is open, this can be mutually beneficial. The teaching agents (school and field instructor) gain the satisfaction of having achieved their own teaching goals and having made their contributions to student progress, client welfare and long term care.

Sensitive Areas

First, is there mutual respect among agency, school and student? Do the agency and school accept each other in their respective roles? Sometimes these two agents are not completely accepting of each other; sometimes they are highly critical. It behooves them to be aware of their interaction and cooperate constructively in their mutual endeavor: student education. A cynical or less than honest relationship is not conducive to the required learning/teaching environment.

Second, if school and agency are not in agreement about student-related issues, what vehicles for constructive intervention are built into the situation? Field instructor and faculty advisor must be able to work things out.

Third, is there open communication with the student? Does the student feel free to share problems with the field instructor, or does the student feel compelled to turn to the faculty advisor (or vice versa)? Are problems taken to school by the student as complaints or points of frustration? Again, this model suggests that built-in communication precludes such a possibility in most cases.

Fourth, what about the matter of student confidentiality? The student should be able to discuss problems of the agency at school or with faculty advisor. This should not be found threatening by the field instructor. Similarly, the student should be able to discuss school situations with the field instructor. Such communication is possible when all agents believe they are cooperating, rather than competing, in a true educational process wherein all are learning. School-agency relationships have been formalized in several different ways: e.g., school recognition of the contribution of the agency and field instructor in the learning/teaching process; school-agency conferences to discuss general matters of mutual concern; and sharing of educational materials and plans between school and field. Both agents should be on the constant lookout for ways of sharing information and developing mutual views regarding the learning process.

Finally, the question of student assignment is sometimes a sensitive one. Does the agency see the student as just another pair of hands in a more-often-than-not understaffed situation? The student's learning environment must be protected jealously by the field instructor, yet there must be some understanding on the part of the student and the school that the agency and its clients must profit in some way from the student's presence. The student's primary goal of learning must be achieved through some act of giving, to both agency and clients. This approach has never failed to enhance the student's learning, to benefit clients and to generate enriched relationships. In summation, all participants in the field experience profit from this model.

Training for Community Programs

K. Della Ferguson, PhD

While most of the preceding papers have addressed direct service models and training students to deliver services, this presentation focuses on training the largest long term care group in the country — family caregivers — and on preparing students as future trainers of these vital links in the service chain.

For some seven years, a coalition in the Utica/Rome area of New York State called PACE (Planning, Advocacy and Coordination for the Elderly in Oneida County) comprising representatives from service agencies and professionals in the area, has been offering a free program to the community twice a year. Originally entitled "Care for Your Aging Parent," the program was renamed "Health for Families of the Aged," when it was discovered that children are not the only caregivers. Utica and Rome are about 15 miles apart, so the program alternates between the two locations: in the fall it is in the Utica area and in the spring, in the Rome area. There are divisions and controversies, not only among those receiving services but also among those providing services.

The training program consists of six sessions and has evolved over the years to meet particular needs. The first two sessions present basic information about aging, because many caregivers are very troubled and worried about changes that are, in fact, quite normal in the aging process. Conversely, other changes that the caregivers seem not to notice may indeed indicate that some intervention is called for. Thus, the first session covers biological changes with aging, taught by a biologist/gerontologist and a nutritionist from the Oneida County Area Agency on Aging. The second session is on normal psychological and behavioral changes and common pathologies in the later years that is taught by the author and a community mental health nurse from the local mobile geriat-

81

ric team. The third session, always popular, is "Cutting the Red Tape." It consists of a panel of representatives from the Social Security Office, the legal aid society and the Department of Social Services, plus a discharge planner and an insurance representative. The fourth session is entitled "The Medical Model" and is presented by a panel that includes the director of the Visiting Nurse Association; the heads of family practice and dental residency programs that have gerontological components in a local hospital; a representative from a local pharmaceutical society; and a podiatrist. The fifth session, entitled "The Aging Network, Part I," includes the director of the Oneida County Area Agency on Aging, plus representatives from CASA, an information and referral service of a local program resource center for independent living that deals with all kinds of handicapping situations, and a director of a local long term care facility. The last session, "Aging Network, Part II," consists of a voluntary action director, the director of the local hospice, the president of the ADRDA (Alzheimer's Disease and Related Disorders Association) local chapter and a senior center director.

The purpose of involving such a diversity of service providers and agency representatives is that this program has proven to serve as an entry point into the system for many people in the community. Because the sessions are well-advertised in newspapers and newsletters and are held in senior centers in the two communities, they attract many attenders who are not connected to the aging network in any way. Further, attendance increases as the program progresses: whereas the first session might draw 20 people, there may be 75 or 80 attending the last session; many of the later joiners are friends and family of the earlier attenders. It is thus very important to have participating agencies represented by significant staff members who can not only explain the services provided but be an identifiable name and face for those who may need to contact a particular agency or program. It is important to note that no panelist or presenter is paid; all participation is completely voluntary.

Each session is scheduled to run from 7:00 to 9:00 p.m.; however, sessions rarely end before 10:30 — the questions go on and on. Many attenders find their need for information is not always immediate, but rather in anticipation of future situations with which they will have to cope. Knowing whom to contact for needed services and assistance relieves a great deal of the anxiety and stress associated with caregiving. This program may not be unique, but there certainly are not enough of them, particularly in rural areas like Oneida County, where resources are more dispersed than they are in urban communities and where the proportion of elderly may be abnormally high (30% in Oneida County) because of the out-migration of younger people in search of employment. Effective network-building is particularly challenging under these circumstances: public transportation is non-existent, poverty is prevalent; services are not easy to access; and the elderly are frequently isolated. The implications for the training of long term care professionals are clear: learning how to serve rural (or even semi-rural) communities must be an integral part of the curriculum. Bringing together the representatives of regional agencies may be a formidable task, but the success of programs such as Oneida County's PACE is evidence of both the need and the rewards: the benefits to caregivers, elderly as well as middle-aged, are enormous.

Outpatient Programs from the Training Point of View: Geriatric Dentistry Training at Columbia University

Lynn Tepper, EdD

For the purposes of this presentation, geriatric dentistry refers to that portion of the pre-doctoral educational curriculum teaching management of the older dental patient. The word geriatric has no specific age assignment; rather, it refers to a time when "social, psychological or biological changes associated with aging impair the full and adequate function of the individual" (American Association of Dental Education).

The geriatric dentistry program, begun in 1982 with a $500,000, 5-year grant at the Columbia University School of Dental and Oral Surgery is designed to prepare dental students to deal effectively and compassionately with the medical, psychological, social and economic concerns of elderly patients, as they affect dental treatment. The program gives students the opportunity to work directly, as members of a multidisciplinary team treating elderly patients, with both well and compromised seniors.

The didactic components of the program have been integrated into the second and third years of the curriculum, with special clinical application in year four. A total of seven lectures on geriatric issues are integrated into courses such as "Human Growth and Development" and "Introduction to the Patient, I" in year two. Six additional lectures are given in year three, as part of the course "Introduction to Geriatric Dentistry." In a weekly senior practice seminar, taken in year four, students are required to apply the didactic material from years two and three to actual cases they see.

Dental education in general is quite time-consuming. Students in the first two years spend about 38 hours a week in lectures and laboratories (some five hours a week more than medical students). Thus, finding room in this very crowded curriculum for lectures on geriatrics has been a serious challenge. The author, who does most of this geriatric teaching, had to negotiate with instructors for isolated, scattered hours in the courses that now include her lectures. She was also able to develop the course "Introduction to the Patient," essentially about behavioral sciences, which she directs as well and in which several Division of Geriatrics and Gerontology faculty (e.g., Patricia Miller and Shura Saul) serve as guest lecturers to infuse geriatric content.

EDUCATIONAL OBJECTIVES

Students who have completed the new geriatric dental curriculum are expected to have developed

1. an orientation to the psychosocial aspects of caring for the elderly (more than 50% of the geriatric dental education curriculum deals with other than dental aspects of aging);
2. the ability to consult and work with other professionals involved in treatment of geriatric patients;
3. an ability to design optimal treatment strategies that take into account the multiple behavioral, social, economic and medical problems of both the well and compromised elderly; and
4. the skill to render dental care and dental health instruction to elderly patients as appropriate.

Geriatric Evaluation Group

The Geriatric Evaluation Group (GEG), consisting of a dentist, dental hygienist, social worker and gerontologist, works with students in the clinic as well as in small seminar groups, to provide them with an opportunity, as members of an ongoing health care group, to participate in designing the treatment most appropriate for each geriatric patient.

The major emphasis in the GEG is on helping students acquire and maintain communication skills suited to treating elderly patients. Program faculty feel that the lack of such skills, and the resulting unease caused by dentists' awareness of this lack, are now major barriers to treatment of older patients. The hesitancy is communicated to patients, who are then subtly discouraged from seeking or continuing treatment. A vicious cycle is thus set up: practitioners feel unsuccessful with such patients, adding to insecurity about treating them, and thereby become even more hesitant about accepting elderly patients in the future. The Columbia teaching program is designed to prevent this cycle from the start.

MULTIDISCIPLINARY COLLABORATION

What makes Columbia's geriatric dentistry program unique is the team approach mentioned earlier. This team, consisting of a dentist, social worker, gerontologist and dental hygienist, works chairside in the clinic, as well as with small groups of students, and enables students to learn first-hand that they are members of a team of health professionals who must collaborate with each other in order to provide older patients with the most comprehensive services possible. The team's functions include

1. evaluating patients in the program (often done in the waiting room) to help remove barriers to care;
2. assisting students in planning clinical treatment (treatment approval must come from a dentist, plus another member of the team);
3. helping students prepare comprehensive case presentations (required of all seniors);
4. participating in clinical case conferences (a team member sits in whenever elderly patients are presented);
5. administering the Geriatric Evaluation Survey (described below) to each elderly patient entering the program (done chairside with students); and
6. helping students understand patient concerns and the cooperation necessary between elderly patients and health care providers, if optimum treatment is to be provided.

Team Members' Responsibility

Each member of the multidisciplinary team has clearly defined tasks. They are as follows:

The *dentist* organizes and sequences material for didactic courses, is responsible for liaison with the Associate Dean for Academic Affairs, and, in concert with representatives of the clinical dentistry divisions, supervises clinical dentistry treatment.

The *gerontologist* monitors and evaluates a number of important dimensions of patient-student interactions: attitudinal orientation of students toward patients; ease of interaction; clarity of verbal communication; frequency, quality and appropriateness of touching behaviors that occur; students' ability to pace procedures appropriately; extent of personalization of student-patient encounters through use of patients' names and other techniques; and use of other cues to enhance student-patient interaction.

The *social worker* collaborates with other team members in helping dental students understand the impact of environment on elderly patients' ability to use dental services; and provides information and referral services to elderly patients and their families, particularly when psychosocial and economic problems interfere with patients' ability to make full use of services provided through the program or cause patients to miss clinic appointments.

The *dental hygienist* (manager) assigns patients to dental students; makes appointments for all patients for clinical sessions, in consultation with students; and maintains case progress records on all patients, based on original treatment plans and work completed.

Geriatric Evaluation Survey

This assessment tool was developed specifically for use in the geriatric dentistry training program. Through interviews, it gathers demographic data, as well as information about psychosocial needs and existing (and potential) barriers to care. The survey is administered to each elderly patient in the program by one of the multidisciplinary team members in the presence of the patient's student clinician, who then uses the information in formulating his/her required case presentation.

The success of the geriatric dentistry program at Columbia's

School of Dental and Oral Surgery is nicely reflected by changes observed in dental students by the author. Before the program was instituted, students in the fourth year practice seminar were likely to refer to their patients merely as procedures ("Mrs. T. is a 78-year-old CD/CD with extensive bone resorption . . ."). At a recent practice seminar, one student presented his case thus: "Mrs. M. is an 82-year-old retired chorus girl from the Cotton Club . . ." It is evident that the dental students now can see their elderly patients as individuals rather than just required procedures.

Outpatient Programs from the Training Point of View: Geriatric Medical Training at Columbia University

Lucien Cote, MD

It is most regrettable that the medical school does not have a full-time geriatrician. Most medical practitioners here feel they are at least part-time geriatricians simply because so many of their patients are 65 or older.

Nor does the medical school offer any specific course, or courses, in geriatric medicine. Students get fragmented education in this discipline through isolated lectures in such courses as abnormal human biology and neuroscience (the author lectures on aging of the brain in the latter). Ideally, the medical school would have a full-time geriatrician who could integrate geriatrics into the medical school education and orient students to this specialized area of knowledge.

There is another approach, of perhaps more value, exemplified by an experience the author had in 1984. A medical student discovered that year he could get a small grant ($500 annually) to follow a patient with Alzheimer's disease and asked the author to be his mentor during this study. It was a most valuable experience for both mentor and student. The student met with the patient's family once or twice a week and became like an adopted son to them. The student then met with his mentor about once a month and was able to share insights that practicing physicians usually cannot see because of the normal brevity of contact between doctor and patient.

This may in fact be the ideal model for teaching medical students to deal with the elderly: assign each student a geriatric patient, one

91

chronically ill with, e.g., Alzheimer's or Parkinson's, at the beginning of his/her medical education and have the student work one-to-one with the patient and family for the duration. Indeed, this approach is used by other medical schools in the country, with great success. One hopes that the College of Physicians & Surgeons at Columbia University will consider adopting the model.

The Continuum of Long Term Care: An Educational Guide for Faculty in the Health Sciences

John Toner, EdD

INTRODUCTION

Long Term Care (LTC) refers to a range of health and supportive services for individuals who have lost some capacity for self-care due to a chronic illness or condition and who are expected to need care for an extended period. Long term care services can be provided either formally—by individuals or agencies who are paid for their services, or informally—by relatives or others who provide the services without compensation. The theoretical framework for the development of formal and primary group services to the elderly will make up part of the introduction to this guide. Although this guide is designed to provide an overview of the key information to be incorporated in any curriculum which focuses on the continuum of long term care, more extensive teaching notes and bibliographic information, including appendices which correspond with the session notes, can be obtained by contacting the author directly.

The guide is organized into six major sub-topics which relate directly to the topic of the Continuum of Long Term Care. Each sub-topic is designed to be a formal, didactic session with students at the graduate level or professional staff in medical or allied health fields. The author gratefully acknowledges the support of the American Association of University Programs in Health Administration in the preparation of this guide.

© 1990 by The Haworth Press, Inc. All rights reserved.

SESSION 1:
INTRODUCTION AND OVERVIEW OF LTC

This session addresses a number of issues pertaining to community-based and institutional services available to elderly individuals including health, housing, volunteer and social services. In the context of this module, long term care services are defined as those services whose purpose is to provide preventative, therapeutic, rehabilitative, supportive and maintenance activities for people over the age of 65, who have a chronic physical or mental impairment. (See HCFA reading, Section I and II for a discussion of the rationale for long term care services as well as family vs. public involvement in long term care. HCFA Section II defines long term care, introduces the concept of "functional disability" as it relates to the need for long term care, and describes the characteristics of elderly who are most needy of long term care services). The session will be structured so that the continuum of services is identified by the settings and array of services from the least restrictive to the most restrictive. (See Brody and Maschiocchi article and accompanying Flow Chart, which is cited at the end of this chapter, for a review of the service continuum.) Long term care constitutes a wide variety of services offered in diverse settings to individuals with differing needs and preferences. The continuum stretches from total institutional care in hospitals to a variety of social services to the patient in his/her own home, with a large number of services in between. Ideally, LTC services begin with efforts to prevent deterioration or dependency and end only after ensuring that death and associated suffering have been made as bearable as possible.

The instructor should begin by addressing the need for long term care and how this has often been confused with the need for formal services. The presence or absence of informal support as well as the presence of a disabling acute or chronic condition in large part determines the need for formal support services. Despite its importance to an increasing number of people, LTC remains misunderstood. The evolving concept of the continuum considers long term care needs as varied and changing, and not limited to the patients who receive formal services from nursing homes, out-patient departments of hospitals and physician's offices (i.e., medical settings). The concept of a continuum of long term care services evolves from policy, which itself is determined by legislation (e.g., Older Americans Act and Social Security Amendments). The government's responsibility is to carry out the law. The fact remains, however, that in reality a continuum of coordinated services for the elderly does not exist in this country and probably will never be achieved without the intervention of the government.

The complex and interrelated scope of long term care encompasses health, health-related and social care services. No one definition of LTC is universally accepted. The long term care population includes the impaired chronically ill who need assistance in activities of daily living and residents in LTC institutions, e.g., the aged and a large proportion of younger patients suffering mental retardation.

Although long term care services range along a continuum of required services, public programs disproportionately support institutional care, notably nursing home care. The HCFA report indicates that *less than 10 percent of public funds are devoted to home-based services*. While many disabled receive no long term care, there is evidence that 20 to 40 percent of the nursing home population could be cared for at less intensive levels if adequate community-based care was available. If the instructor wishes, he/she can describe the studies of institutionalized elderly reporting large percentages of unmarried and/or childless residents who lack sufficient community supports.

The three main characteristics of the current LTC services provision are (1) it is dominated by the Medicaid program which stresses medical and institutional care rather than community-based social and support services for people with chronic impairments; (2) it is represented by fragmented federal programs, which inadequately assess needs of persons requiring long term care. Each program deals only with an isolated aspect of an individual's need, e.g., the Supplemental Security Income (SSI) program raises income above the poverty level but neglects to address the issue of quality of life beyond that; and (3) Title III of the Older Americans Act and Title XX of the Social Security Act have provided opportunities for developing community-based services, but neither has achieved the volume of services or the specific focus on LTC which might make such services a major element in the delivery of long term care.

The instructor should also review briefly the financing of LTC. In this regard the Armour, Estes and Noble (1981) and the Ruchlin and Levey (1976) articles will be useful. Current federal programs finance a variety of long term care services at the local level, primarily under Titles XVIII, XIX and XX of the Social Security Act (Medicare, Medicaid and Social Services), and Title III of the Older Americans Act (Social and Nutrition Services and Senior Centers). Medicaid, Title XX and Title III are state-administered, while Medicare is federally-administered. Income maintenance is provided mainly through Social Security, i.e., Old Age, Survivors and Disability Insurance and the Supplemental Security Income program which are federally-administered. Housing-oriented programs are operated by the Department of Housing and Urban Development, often under state and local administration. Although these programs contribute to meeting long term care needs, the system emphasizes health services because that is where federal financial support is concentrated.

While present programs are not comprehensive nor uniform across states, all states cover some range of services critically important to the health and continued independence of many chronically impaired persons. Medicaid coverage, for example, does not extend to all elderly poor in need of these services. Since each state has some discretion in setting its eligibility standards, the resulting variation contributes to the inequities of the system.

The session also focuses on disability and chronic illness and definitions of disability, impairment and handicap in the elderly. (See Cole article.) Finally, the session also deals with prevalence and significance of disability as it relates to the community, home-bound, hospitalized and nursing home elderly (see HCFA, pp. 3-16). The instructor should review the HCFA article and devote time to the definition and measurement of "functional disability" and Tables II-1 to II-2. The instructor should discuss these prevalence estimates and their significance in the development of services in the LTC continuum. The session should also review the normal physical and biological changes associated with aging, age-related changes in the major organ systems and survey the diseases commonly associated with aging. To this end, the Saxon and Etten book, which is a concise, readable and applied review and was written for students who do not have basic science backgrounds, and the Pizer book, which emphasizes the diseases commonly associated with older age as well as other health related topics, may be used. Either at the end of the session or as a take-home assignment, students can complete the Palmore Facts on Aging Quiz and either discuss it in class or incorporate their reaction to the quiz in their session critique.

Cole's article focuses on the concepts of disability and rehabilitation and their implications for elderly populations. The session should stress that disability is a very instrumental factor in determining whether or not a person seeks long term care.

A distinction should also be made among the concepts of impairment, disability and handicap. Impairment is an abnormal physiological or mental process that occurs within an individual. Disability is the physical manifestation of such abnormality. Handicaps are the effects that these manifestations have upon the individual in question, that is, whether these manifestations limit the person in a function deemed crucial in his or her life. According to some definitions, disability and subsequent handicap both imply chronic conditions, those that last longer than three months, rather than acute conditions.

Fifteen percent of the U.S. population are handicapped due to a disability and of this percentage, the elderly constitute the greatest proportion. Although age and disability are directly proportional, most aged persons do not become handicapped until they reach the "frail elderly" stage, which begins at 85. Recent studies indicate that more than 34% of those over the age of 85 require assistance in performing at least one Activity of Daily Living (ADL), such as dressing or bathing, and 39% of this age group require assistance in performing at least one instrumental (IADL) such as shopping. This is a substantial increase from the population between the ages of 75 and 84, in which only about 11% and 14.2% require assistance in ADL and IADL, respectively. Therefore, the older one gets, the greater the chances that one will spend the rest of one's life unable to perform both basic and instrumental activities of daily living. It is when the individual becomes completely dependent on others for activities of daily living that long term care is initiated.

Rehabilitation is considered the final phase of the medical care continuum, following prevention and acute care. Rehabilitation seeks to improve the quality of one's life by optimizing abilities. In a sense, rehabilitation is prevention, in that it can restore an individual's capacity to perform all types of activities of daily living, which would in turn prevent the individual from seeking long term care. Thus, rehabilitation could in some cases allow the individual to remain in the community and function independently. Considering the costs of long term institutionalization and home care services, rehabilitation services could become an instrumental facet of long term care policy in the future.

In addition to its potential monetary benefits, rehabilitation also is beneficial by definition. As human beings, as living organisms, we all strive to maintain our optimal state of existence. Rehabilitation could mean the difference between dependency and independence, and institutionalization.

SESSION 2:
THE EVOLUTION OF LTC SERVICES

This session begins with an introduction to the history of growth and development of long term care in the United States. The instructor and students should describe their own backgrounds and experience in long term care in order to provide a framework for discussion of the Benjamin article, the Moroney article and the Vogel and Palmer chapters.

The instructor should review the Benjamin article with the intention of discussing its contents with students. No more than 15 minutes of the session should be devoted to the review of this material. The Moroney and Kurtz article can then serve as a framework for a 20-30 minute discussion of the evolution of long term care institutions, and the instructor should be careful to delineate the periods of development as described by Moroney and Kurtz.

The Moroney and Kurtz chapter describes the growth and development of long term care in America. The history of this growth seems to be unique to the U.S. There is also an attempt to predict the future of long term care in America.

The authors employ a "systems analysis" approach in examining the place of long term care in America. Four assumptions are made in a systems analysis:

1. The total system has a goal that is common to its sub-systems.
2. The sub-systems are interdependent.
3. Functions develop within the system in response to the needs of the system.
4. No single part or sub-system completely controls the whole system. The authors think that such an analysis of long term care will help identify strengths and weaknesses of linkages between the units that comprise the *total system* or goal.

A systems analysis required a clear statement of goals. There are four goals for the larger health care system in this country: prevention of disease; treatment of disease; rehabilitation of patients; and maintenance. Obviously long term care is a sub-system of total health care whose primary goal is *maintenance*, although the other 3 goals may at times be involved in long term care.

The authors next undertake an historical analysis of care of the aged in the Western world. In Greek and Roman times the disabled and aged were considered a drain on society and so "abandonment" was often practiced. With the appearance of Christianity, caring for the sick was seen as the exercise of charity that could gain spiritual reward for the caretakers. This type of church-sponsored care reached its peak in the Middle Ages. In the 17th century in England, "Poor Laws" were passed. Under this plan, parishes put able bodied paupers to work and provided a place of habitation for the needy and elderly who were unable to work. If the needy or elderly had relatives who could provide "support" they could not enter the system. This pauper system lasted into the 19th century. Thus the impoverished elderly often ended up in "almshouses" along with the insane, feebleminded, epileptics, blind and deaf mutes, sufferers of chronic diseases, criminals, prostitutes, mothers of illegitimate children, orphans and deserted children. In colonial America care of the elderly followed the English mode.

The modern period includes four sub-periods.

1. *1900-1935*. The twentieth century received a troublesome legacy of mistreatment and neglect of the elderly. The Charitable Organization Society moved to get the aged out of the public almshouses and to eliminate the need for public administration of relief. Efforts were made to develop a system of privately financed boarding homes. In 1910 the Flexner reports resulted in a marked improvement in physician training and in better standards of medical care. These efforts at improvement were directed toward acute care in hospitals rather than to long term care. The Great Depression, with its many poor people of all ages, brought to the hospitals great financial difficulty. Boarding homes had been established for the elderly, but in this era they were outside of the medical system. Voluntary health insurance to help with high medical costs began to appear and was looked at with great interest by the financially "strapped" hospitals. During this period the primary source of health care was the physicians who determined the place and course of treatment for elderly patients.

2. *1935-1949*. The two most important changes affecting the linkage of health care sub-systems were the expansion of voluntary health insurance and the advent of the Social Security Act of 1935. The health sub-systems linkage remained much the same as in the earlier era. The trend continued to center all medical care around the hospital. Boarding homes and convalescent homes became more popular as modes of care for the elderly. Because they did not wish to lose large numbers of sick elderly people, some of the homes began to provide nursing services and some of the boarding homes thus evolved into *nursing homes*. However, these "nursing homes" were not integrated into the medical care system.

3. *1950-1964*. During this period there was a marked increase in the numbers of elderly persons requiring health care. Chronically ill, elderly patients were filling acute-care beds in hospitals. The hospitals themselves began to look for means to ease this overcrowding. Health insurance continued to expand until in 1960, 87% of the total population had some hospital coverage. However, in the

high-risk group (those over age 65), only about 47% were covered. Government intervention appeared to be necessary. A most dramatic change for the elderly had occurred with the passage of the Social Security Act of 1935. In this Act were included Old Age Survivors' Insurance (OASI) and Old Age Assistance (OAA). The latter program was administered by the federal government and state welfare departments. These programs gave the elderly the choice of remaining in their own homes or going to boarding and convalescent homes, some of which became nursing homes. (Such federal grants were not available to "persons in such public institutions as almshouses or county farms." Therefore, the elderly had little incentive to go to public institutions.) Since 1950 the federal government, modifying its program of cash payments to recipients, has shared in payments which states make directly to vendors (those providing medical services) under OAA. Experience had indicated that cash payments given to the elderly did not satisfactorily cover their medical expenses. States, if they wished, could pay for additional medical services for the aged, but such additional payments were not matched by federal funds. Since 1960 special federal assistance has been available to states spending dollars on medical care for the elderly. Congress passed the legislation, Medical Assistance for the Aged (MAA), and it was known as the Kerr-Mills Bill. This Bill substantially increased federal sharing with states in vendor payments, and states were expected to expand their medical care programs for the aged. However, few states were willing to allocate additional funds for such care programs, even with matching federal monies. Thus a relatively small number of states used the bulk of MAA funds. During this period, hospitals needed nursing homes, although they were reluctant to establish working relationships with them that would imply recognition of their legitimacy. Thus the linkage between hospitals and nursing homes in providing long term care improved.

4. *1965-1972.* In this period efforts were made to bring the nursing home industry into the mainstream of the health care system. The most significant legislation passed was PL89-97 (Medicare and Medicaid), designed to aid medically "high risk groups," the aged and the poor. This legislation made two major assumptions:

— The insurance program would meet the needs of the aged. The welfare component was a secondary program to supplement Medicare to meet the needs of a few individuals. This assumption proved to be erroneous.

— Given financial incentives, the nursing home industry would respond by developing additional resources (it did to some degree) and comply with federal standards for participation (it did *not*).

The second assumption made an attempt to regulate the nursing home industry by certification. By July 1969 the number of fully-certified homes had almost doubled. A demand for nursing home care for the elderly had been created. Politically and socially the government had only one option: to certify nursing homes that failed to meet the "standard" as ECFs (extended care facilities). Costs spiralled. Medicaid faced similar problems. Under Title XIX the federal government agreed to match state payments for care of patients at the level of *skilled nursing homes*. If the patient was classified as in need of a lower level of institutional care, the state was reimbursed at the old standard old-age-assistance rate. With this kind of financial incentive, some states reclassified lower level facilities to SNFs and as many patients as possible as in need of "skilled nursing care." Thus there was no incentive to lower costs. In 1967 Congress enacted PL 90-248 so that federal matching funds were authorized for a lower level of care in the "intermediate care facility." There was the understanding that as many as 50% of patients in SNFs could in fact have their needs met at the intermediate level. In general the states have made no substantial effort to classify ICFs. Rather than improve care and reduce costs, many states have simply licensed *any* nursing home as an ICF which failed to qualify as a skilled nursing home with a decrease in the level of services provided. The federal government has assumed a central role in the total process of medical care while still adhering to the principle of non-interference (up to 1972). Legislative programs have been disappointing. Despite increased funding, nursing homes did not enthusiastically respond to the opportunities to upgrade services and standards and to extend care.

The Vogel and Palmer chapters can serve as the major material for the balance of the session; Chapter VII of Vogel and Palmer focuses on "the alternatives question." The chapter focuses primarily on costs, cost-effectiveness and cost-efficiency. These issues are extremely controversial, and students should be encouraged to deal with the controversial nature and implications of these concepts in their session critiques. The emphasis should be on the need for looking at costs for given *quality* of care. Indeed, for Pollak (cited in Vogel and Palmer, VII), cost of long term care is a function of care at a given level of quality for a given level of impairment. The instructor should emphasize that the trick is to define and measure quality. In fact, families/patients do not agree with most professionals — according to a study described in the Coe and Kahana chapter — and see less need for services than the professionals do. The two Vogel and Palmer chapters — i.e., Chapter VII (Alternatives) and Chapter X (Housing) — refer to a continuum of long term care facilities and programs. The instructor should point out and define the notion of "crystal lattice" as described in Chapter VII.

Discussion of the development of national, state and local administrative structures for long term care services should precede discussion of the U.S. DHHS channeling initiative.

The final segment of this session should be devoted to a discussion of the National Long Term Care Demonstration (channeling) multistate research experiment. This research program was designed primarily to determine once and for all if community care was a cost-efficient alternative to nursing home care. The three articles from the Health Services Research Journal listed in the readings for Session 2 provide the core of information on the channeling demonstration program. Two of these readings (Carcagno and Kemper, 1988; and Weissert, 1988) are required and contain most of the material which students should master. The instructor should discuss the concept of channeling with particular attention given to the role of basic case management in channeling as well as the financial control model described by Carcagno and Kemper (p.3). Additionally, the instructor should discuss the intended effects of the demonstration program including the increased use of community services, reduced use of nursing homes, reduced use of hospitals and reduced cost of long term care. Finally, the instructor should review with students what was learned from the demonstration and the current focus of research efforts in this area.

SESSION 3:
FAMILY CAREGIVING,
FORMAL AND INFORMAL SUPPORT STRUCTURES

This session is designed to sensitize the student to the multifaceted variables related to the provision of care for the elderly by formal and informal support systems.

The provision of long term care for the elderly presents problems that are complex and multidimensional in nature, e.g., issues of financial, physical and emotional dependence/independence of both the dependent elderly person as well as the caregiver. There are no facile answers or solutions to these issues for either the elderly individual or caregiver. The solutions are often imperfect and frequently as complicated as the problems themselves. The issue of funding for long term care has become more and more current, especially during this election season. A concise report in the (Sunday, February 7, 1988) *New York Times* provides some startling statistics relating to the provision of home health care benefits. A study conducted by the Congressional Budget Office (CBO) relating to administration cuts in home care benefits under Medicare found that "$2.4 billion less was spent on home health and nursing home benefits since 1984 than the amount Congress had estimated was needed. In the same period, studies have shown a doubling of demand for some home health services. The growth rate of home health care coverage plummeted from 20 percent in 1984 and 16.7 percent in 1985 to 4.3 percent in 1986 and 6.4 percent in 1987." The emphasis on cost containment and reduction in services can be found in the CBO's view of the reason for the drop in services, ". . . coverage restrictions imposed by the Health Care Financing Administration."

The instructor should devote at least 10-20 minutes to the distinctions identified by Litwak regarding formal institutions and primary group structures. This will also involve a discussion of the communication gap between the service providers and caregivers. This discussion should be followed by a discussion of the issues regarding family caregiving as delineated in the Treas and Shanas articles.

SESSION 4:
THE CONTINUUM OF LONG TERM CARE SERVICES

The continuum of long term care services is described in this session by a discussion of the primary target populations to be served (e.g., well elderly, temporarily ill elderly, frail elderly residing in the community and frail elderly who are residing in institutions); the types of services available (e.g., nutrition, health/medical, home supports, recreational/educational/social/cultural, mental health, housing, transportation, legal, life management and financial assistance); and the purpose of those services (e.g., preventative, therapeutic, rehabilitative, supportive and maintenance). In this session, the instructor should address a number of issues pertaining to community-based services available to elderly individuals, including health, housing, volunteer and social services. According to the definition cited by Monk, social services can be defined as "a flexibly organized system of activities and institutions to help attain satisfying standards of life and health while helping people develop their full capacities in personal and social relationships." Clearly, this illustrates the value of social service providers with assisting the elderly in maintaining their independence in light of any chronic or functional disabilities they may sustain. Therefore, social service providers must shift from focusing on symptom-oriented treatment to focusing on disease-preventive and health promotional strategies. This shift is imperative in order to encourage the elderly to enhance their health status and develop self-reliance.

Now that the 1982 Tax Equity and Fiscal Responsibility Act (TEFRA) is quite a few years old, problems inherent in parts of this legislation are being identified. In particular, the new classification system based on Diagnosis Related Groups (DRGs) appears to affect adversely the health care services and treatment received by the elderly on Medicare. (The situation is similar for those individuals on Medicaid.) Designed to streamline patient care, DRGs often prompt hospitals to discharge their elderly patients "quicker and sicker" in order to save money. Consequently, it has been shown that early discharge of the elderly results in both a higher utilization rate of skilled nursing facilities, as well as a greater rate of rehospitalization. Aside from the potential abuse of the elderly, DRGs end up costing the elderly more money in the long run. Clearly, this system must be reevaluated in order to provide the elderly with quality health care both in the hospital and within the community.

The instructor should also raise the point that there are few educational/training requirements for those who provide much of the care for the home-bound elderly. Those home care services reimbursable under Medicare and Medicaid are for the most part provided by formal caregivers who are not subject to any formal training or supervision within the different organizations providing this care. The Home and Community Based Services for the Elderly Act of 1985 (Bill S. 1181), which calls for such training of home care personnel providing medical services to the elderly, should be discussed as a possible solution to home care abuses.

A major portion of this session should be devoted to a discussion of the long term care service continuum.

Instructors should use the Evashwick and Plein (1982) monograph for the discussion of health and social service professionals' roles in nursing homes and can engage participants from other settings in a discussion of how the roles of professionals in nursing homes might contrast with the function of corresponding professionals in different settings.

SESSION 5:
MECHANISMS FOR LINKING OLDER PERSONS' NEEDS WITH APPROPRIATE LONG TERM CARE SERVICES AND ASSURING COORDINATION OF SERVICES

This session will be devoted to describing assessment mechanisms for linking client/patient needs to appropriate services along the continuum of long term care. Reliable objective assessment of functional loss is crucial in designing, developing and allocating remedial and restorative services for the elderly. Assessment must include not only careful medical and psychosocial evaluations with special attention to the needs and problems of the elderly, but reasonable objective measures as well. In order to be truly comprehensive, functional assessment must be an interdisciplinary effort utilizing as many reproducible measures as possible.

For the past several years, the author, Dr. Barry Gurland and others at the Center for Geriatrics and Gerontology have been working with the Division of General Medicine at Columbia to develop a systematic interview for elderly patients in primary care medical practice. The interview (the MERGE-CARE) covers problems in a variety of physical, mental, emotional and social functions and is innovatively keyed to decision making (see Toner and Gurland, 1987). The session will include a brief discussion of CARE and MERGE-CARE as examples of methods linking older persons' needs with appropriate long term care services.

SESSION 6:
MODEL LONG TERM CARE SERVICE SYSTEM

There does not yet exist in this country a coordinated system and continuum of care for the elderly, yet the creation of such a system should be a main objective of the organization of services. Achieving this objective will require defining the components of a good system of care, examining examples of successful systems and identifying means of improving, expanding and generalizing these efforts. In this direction an international conference was sponsored by the Center for Geriatrics and Gerontology and held at Columbia University in October, 1986. The author of this chapter was co-chairman of the conference, which stimulated discussion among a select multidisciplinary group concerned with the health of the elderly. The discussion focused on the desirability, feasibility, progress and achievements in building a complete system of health care for the elderly. A major focus of this symposium was cross-national comparison of systems of care. The proceedings of the conference have been published by Springer Publishing as a chapter in *Essentials of Geriatric Psychiatry: A Guide for Health Professionals*, edited by Lawrence Lazarus.

The session will focus on three areas of long term care services: physical health services, social services, and mental health services and will utilize the products of the symposium in reviewing model long term care programs in England and Canada.

Finally, the session will review the impact of various state long term care assessment and service initiatives (as described by Benjamin, 1985), including those of Wisconsin, Connecticut, Oregon, Florida, Minnesota, Massachusetts and New York. This component will include demonstration and/or pilot projects, multiple funding streams, Medicaid waiver opportunities, established statewide networks of agencies, developed or developing strategies for the elderly to get access to services before becoming poor and slotted to institutional care, breakdown of boundaries between acute and long term care through informed discharge planning and prescreening of potential nursing home clients, and the role of hospital planners and client management staff in community care networks.

Different countries have addressed long term care in ways influenced by cultural tradition and social policy. For the sake of comparison, it is useful to look at the development of various "systems" of long term care in the search for improved health and welfare programs and cost-effective strategies, which may be appropriate to the United States system of care to the elderly.

The U.S. spectrum of care presently includes acute care (hospitals), community services (professional and nonprofessional), day care and respite care, with individuals getting a mixture of benefits and services depending upon the economic status and generosity of the state and the facility of a case manager to assign or "broker" these services. Model programs, mostly concerned with issues of service delivery, are underway, but rarely are these connected with other programs. In addition, most long term care strategies fail to account for the individuals as members of family units. New approaches, including the Lombardi program in New York State, multifunctional hospitals (nursing homes) and social HMOs, are also being implemented in an effort to serve long term care needs. In sum, the U.S. nonsystem is fragmented, duplicative and often inaccessible.

With the development of the National Health Service after World War II, England established a range of programs and retirement benefits for their elderly through appropriations to the national budget. In contrast to the situation in the U.S., England placed a high priority on health and social services at the national level and set forth a national plan for such services. Property taxes fund these programs, which are then administered through local authorities (based on geographic areas). The General Practitioner (GP) acts as a "gatekeeper" to community-based services and as a member of the community health care team (social worker, district health nurse, geriatric worker, community psychiatric nurse, MESS squad and home helps). Other community services (day care and meal programs) are available; specialized geriatric hospitals (reserved for acute cases) and geriatric consultants are utilized through referral from the GP. Local authority homes, developed from retirement homes, are administered under the auspices of Social Services (with social workers as matrons). Lacking a medical director and institutional atmosphere, these local authority homes continue to promote the use of the community GP and health care team just as these services are used within the community. However, as the numbers of frail elderly aging increase, there are signs that the local authority homes should move toward becoming more medicalized.

Major Differences/Similarities:
New York and London

The prevalence of dementia is about the same in both cities (40%), with a higher percentage of the care given to demented individuals in New York given in nursing institutions (67%). In London, 64% of the care provided for demented individuals is rendered in residential settings. Moreover, a higher percentage of demented are likely to be in skilled nursing beds in New York (90%). New York facilities for long term care are more "medicalized," having more staff and bigger physical plants, often with demented patients separated or segregated from others, while small, residential facilities, with little segregation of patients and more heterogeneous mix (due largely to the size of the facility) are are found in London. New York appears to devote much more of its health resources to long term institutional care: larger, more sophisticated, more technological and more expensive facilities are the norm, with little data available to suggest that care and/or quality of life is any better for the demented, elderly patient. New York houses 90% demented in institutions whereas London places only 50% in the local authority homes.

The Canadian System

Kane and Kane (1985) discuss the Canadian system. The Canadian system of long term care is an extension of its nationalized program of health insurance which has been in effect for many years. Certain aspects of the Canadian socio-cultural and economic system may have an impact on the nationalized system of long term care. For instance, Canada's population is only ten percent of that of the United States. Its federal system is much smaller with only ten provinces and two territories. This makes health care financing and planning less complex. Fewer hospitals, medical schools and government agencies make coordination of services less cumbersome. Canada has a parliamentary system of government and a greater public acceptance of a large role for government. Since the population of Canada is more homogenous than that of the United States, the delivery of services is much more acceptable to formal service providers and the elderly alike.

The long term care system in Canada uses a mix of for-profit and non-profit provider agencies and institutions. Although a person's income is taken into consideration, every older person is assured nursing home care without means or assets tests. The level of functional impairment is the basis for eligibility. Clients pay a moderate room charge designed to leave even those dependent solely on government pensions with a small discretionary income. Typically, provider facilities are paid on a per diem basis annually negotiated for the whole province, whereas non-profit facilities are on the basis of prospectively negotiated global budgets.

In 1982, public expenditures in Canada per nursing home bed averaged $9,600 in U.S. currency, as compared with combined state and federal expenditures of approximately $10,000 in the United States. In the Canadian provinces, remaining costs are largely financed by user fees paid directly by the consumer (each province establishes a fixed per diem "ward rate" at an amount keyed to the minimum pension). Additional charges for private rooms and specified amenities are permitted but strictly controlled. The highest rate per bed (in the Manitoba province) is $15,400 as compared to the U.S. average of $18,200.

The long term care provisions of three Canadian provinces serve as the central theme of the Kane and Kane (1985) book. The provinces are Ontario, Manitoba and British Columbia. Using the Kane and Kane book, the instructor should briefly describe the salient features of the system in effect in each province. In her unpublished paper, Moss (1987) reviewed the Canadian system of LTC as described by Kane and Kane. According to Kane and Kane (as cited by Moss) in Ontario, there is a fixed daily amount for SNF care ($15.68) which the client has to pay; he or she is then left with approximately $96 of the pension each month for personal expenses.

The instructor should discuss the role of homes for the aged. These homes were started prior to the initiation of the long term care program in Ontario and were established by municipalities or non-profit organizations to provide residential care to senior citizens who could not or preferred not to live in the community. Residents pay according to means, and deficits the homes incur are met by the sponsoring organization or municipality and the province. There are now 13,000 persons in extended care beds in homes for the aged. These clients cannot pay the customary user charge, but the home is reimbursed for the actual expenses incurred because the Government picks up the deficit. Ontario also has chronic care hospitals which also provide long term care. Some may be free-standing but the majority are usually sections of general hospitals. These beds are paid for as part of the hospitals' global budget from the province and are free to its users. However, after the 60th day, all residents in such hospitals (and all residents in acute care hospitals awaiting a lower level of care) are assigned the $15.68 daily residential charge.

Since 1968 Ontario has had a medically oriented acute home care program as part of its insurance benefit. It includes nursing and therapeutic services and a maximum of eighty hours of homemaking per admission. Ontario's program of chronic home care was introduced as a pilot program in 1975, and as of 1984 has been in full swing, covering all 38 health districts. It provides 80 hours of homemaking in the first month and 40 hours in each subsequent month per admission, assuming that at least three visits per month were required for professional care. The province is considering a homemaking service benefit for those not requiring professional home care. Home care in Ontario is free. The amount given to each client is determined by home care case managers located in each health district. The Ministry of Health purchases nursing services from voluntary agencies at rates negotiated on a provincial level; homemaking services are purchased from non-profit or proprietary agencies. Although home care case managers have a sharply limited role, they represent a major source for rationalizing home-based services. Some districts in Ontario have placement coordinators who complete assessments of all extended care applicants in their assigned districts and manage a centralized waiting list of these patients.

Manitoba has four levels of nursing home care going from level one, for those patients who require no more than 30 minutes of nursing care per day, to level four, which is analogous to Ontario's chronic care hospitals and is also offered in extended care units of general hospitals.

Since 1975 community care and case-management services in Manitoba have been provided by continuing care programs housed in each local health and social services department. Nurse-social worker teams serve as continuing care coordinators who assess eligibility for all long term care services, including SNF care, home care and day care. Homemaking is provided directly by public employees, up to the maximum number of hours authorized by the coordinators. Nursing and therapies are provided directly also, but may be purchased from non-profit agencies as well.

No person may enter a SNF without the case being reviewed by an interdisciplinary panel. Home care coordinators are responsible for assessing the applicants to SNFs, organizing the information for the panel hearings, and managing the waiting list of persons who have been accepted for facilities. The panel reviews medical information (from the applicant's own physician) as well as social information, which helps to decide the appropriate plan for the individual patient. Home care expenditures per client are limited to those for a nursing home patient at the same level — exceptions are made for short-term terminal care if an SNF bed is available. Applicants are encouraged to make their own first and second choices of facilities. If forced to enter a different facility to free a hospital bed, they are put on the waiting list for the facility of their choice.

In British Columbia there are five levels of nursing home care including a personal care level, three intermediate care levels and one extended care level for those who are unable to get out of bed independently. British Columbia is divided into districts which administer long term care benefits. In each district, managers assess the functional status of applicants and determine their level of care. Case managers may authorize homemaker services up to maximum limits set for each level of care; they may also authorize day care. Homemaker services are purchased from non- and for-profit agencies. Home nursing visits are provided by nurses from the public health departments. Case managers review each case every six months, after every intervening hospitalization or as requested by the client or care provider. Case managers continue to follow up their assessments of the patients' needs no matter what kind of long term care they are receiving. As long term care benefits have been introduced over the past decade in various provinces, the rate of health care spending in Canada, expressed as a proportion of the GNP, has remained consistently below that of the U.S. Moss (1987) also summarizes the lessons to be learned from Canada's nationalized system of long term care. These lessons can be used in the development of a national system of long term care in the United States. A national system jointly financed by the federal and state governments, with each state government administering its own program, might be a productive solution. Each state must accept the same long term care program which has been devised and approved by the Senate, the House of Representatives and the President of the United States. Each state would be divided into geographical units or districts, each with a public health department which would strictly and conscientiously determine the long term care needs of each candidate who came before it, with respect to his or her medical and social needs. There would be case managers to monitor the progress and on-going needs of each patient in the long term and to adjust the plans for the patient accordingly. There should be no means testing of the elderly in order to gain access to the system; all should be eligible for these long term care services. In addition to joint federal and state funding, a certain portion of the elderly's monthly pension should be withheld for use by the government in the continued financing of long term care.

The idea of a national system of long term care in the United States is a very exciting one, but one that can become a reality only if Americans and the American government come to realize that good health care is a right, not a privilege.

NOTE: The list of references that follows is specific to this instruction module. The references marked with asterisks are those thought to be most central to session discussion.

LIST OF REFERENCES

Session 1:
Introduction and Overview of Long Term Care

*Flow Chart, Continuum of Long Term Care Services. From article.

Brody, S. J., & Maschiocchi, C. (1980). Data for long term care planning by health system agencies. *American Journal of Public Health*, *70*, 1194-1198.

*Health Care Financing Administration. (January 1981). Long term care: Background and future directions. Section II.

Hudson, R. (1981). The "graying" of the federal budget and its consequences for old-age policy. In R. Hudson (ed.), *The aging in politics, policy, and process* (Ch. 15, pp. 261-281). Springfield, IL: Charles C. Thomas.

*Cole, P. (1979). Morbidity in the United States. In E. Jaco (ed.), *Patients, physicians and illness*. New York: Free Press.

Saxon, S. & Etten, M. (1987). *Physical change and aging*. New York: Teresias Press.

Pizer, H. (ed.) (1985). *Over fifty-five, healthy and alive*. New York: Van Nostrand Reinhold.

Session 2:
The Evolution of Long Term Care Services

*Coe, R. & Kahana, E. (1976). Alternatives in long term care. In S. Sherwood (ed.), *Long term care: A handbook for researchers, planners and providers*. New York: Spectrum Publications, Inc.

HCFA, Section III (B & C), Section IV (B & C), Section V (E & F).

*Benjamin, Jr., A. E. (1985). Community-based long term care. In

C. Harrington, R. Newcome, C. Estes & Associates (eds.), *Long term care of the elderly* (Ch. 9, pp. 197-211). Beverly Hills: Sage Publications.

*Carcagno, G. & Kemper, P. (1988). The evaluation of the national long term care demonstration: An overview of the Channeling Demonstration and its evaluation. *Health Services Research*, *23*, 1-23.

Kemper, P. (1988). The evaluation of the national long term care demonstration: Overview of the findings. *Health Services Research*, *23*, 161-174.

*Weissert, W. (1988). The National Channeling Demonstration: What we knew, know now, and still need to know. *Health Services Research*, *23*, 175-187.

*Moroney, R. & Kurtz, N. (1976). The evaluation of long term care institutions. In S. Sherwood (ed.), *Long term care: A handbook for researchers, planners and providers* (pp. 81-116). New York: Spectrum Publications.

*HCFA, Section III A.

Vogel, R. J. & Palmer, H. C. (eds.) (1985). *Long term care perspectives from research and demonstration* (Chapters XII and X). Rockville: Aspen Systems Corporation.

Monk, A. (ed.) (1985). *Handbook of gerontological services*. New York: Van Nostrand Reinhold.

Session 3:
Family Caregiving, Formal and Informal Support Structures

*Monk, A. (1979). Family supports in old age. *Social Work, November*, 533-538.

*Bennett, R. (1983). Care of the demented: LTC institution, home and family care. In R. Mayeux & W. Rosen (eds.), *The dementias*. New York: Raven Press.

Estes, C., Gerard, L. & Stone, R. (1986). The policy implications of caring for older women. *Business and Health, March*, 38-40.

Shanas, E. (1979). The family as a social support system in old age. *The Gerontologist*, *19* (2), 169-174.

Sangl, J. A. (1985). Family networks. In R. Vogel & H. Palmer (eds.), *Long term care perspectives from research and demonstration* (Ch. VIII). Rockville, MD: Aspen Systems Corporation.

Treas, J. (1977). Family support systems for the aged: Some social and demographic considerations. *The Gerontologist, 17* (6), 486-491.

Young, Jr., W. M. (1982, August). *Family support and the elderly*. New York: Columbia University, Brookdale Collection on Gerontology, Bibliographic Series, No. 8.

Session 4:
The Continuum of Long Term Care Services

*Monk, A. (ed.) (1985). *Handbook of gerontological services* (Ch. 1, pp. 12-38; Ch. 2-3). New York: Van Nostrand Reinhold.

*Evashwick, C. & Plein, J. (eds.) (1982). *Health and social service professionals in nursing homes*. A monograph produced by the Interdisciplinary Nursing Home Program, University of Washington, Long Term Care Gerontology Center, Seattle, Washington.

Session 5:
Mechanisms for Linking Older Persons' Needs
with Appropriate Long Term Care Services
and Assuring Coordination of Services

*Kane, R. A. & Kane, R. L. (1981). *Assessing the elderly* (Ch. 1, pp. 1-23). Lexington, MA: Lexington Books.

*Crook, T. (1979). Psychometric assessment in the elderly. In A. Raskin & L. Jarvik (eds.), *Psychiatric symptoms and cognitive loss in the elderly* (pp. 207-220). New York: Hemisphere Publishing Co.

Brocklehurst, J. C. (1973). *Textbook of geriatric medicine and gerontology* (Ch. 3, pp. 47-57; Ch. 23, pp. 744-749). London: Churchill Livingstone.

Plutchik, R. (1980). Conceptual and practical issues in the assessment of the elderly. In A. Raskin & L. Jarvik (eds.), *Psychiatric symptoms and cognitive loss in the elderly*. New York: Hemisphere Publishing Co.

Sheehan, S. (1983). *Is there no place on earth for me?* New York: Vintage Press.

*Toner, J. (1982) The process of assessment. Charts. (See Teaching Notes.)

*Toner, J. & Gurland, B. (1987). The CARE Interview: An efficient, systematic, multidimensional tool to measure health status of older people. In G. Maddox & E. Busse (eds.), *Aging: The universal human experience, highlights of the 1985 International Congress of Gerontology*. New York: Springer Publishing Co.

Session 6:
Model Long Term Care Service Systems

*Kane, R. A. & Kane, R. L. (1985). *A will and a way: What the United States can learn from Canada about caring for the elderly* (Ch. 3, pp. 75-84 and 103-105; Ch. 4, pp. 106-113 and 130-132; Ch. 5, pp. 140-169, Ch. 9). New York: Columbia University Press.

Kane, R. A. & Kane, R. L. (1985). The feasibility of universal long term care benefits: Ideas from Canada. *New England Journal of Medicine, 312,* 1357-1364.

*Gurland, B., Toner, J., Mustille, A. et al. (1988). The organization of mental health services for the elderly. In L. Lazarus (ed.), *Essentials of geriatric psychiatry* (pp. 189-213). New York: Springer Publishing Company.

Reinhard, S. (1986). Financing long term health care of the elderly: Dismantling the medical model. *Public Health Nursing, 3,* 3-22.

PART III:
POLICIES FOR DEVELOPMENT OF SUCCESSFUL MODELS: PAST, PRESENT AND FUTURE

Introduction to Part III

Currently, most of community-based long term care, whether successful or unsuccessful, is determined by public funding streams stemming from counties, municipalities, states and the federal government. These funding streams are determined by public policy: at times the public is generous towards the elderly; at other times, the social climate shifts and other groups are seen to be more "deserving." Needless to say, such shifts can wreak havoc at the local level where many elderly may be fully dependent on comprehensive programs and benefits, without which they could no longer reside in the community.

Thus, it is important for the elderly as well as for all people, including students, to understand public policies and how they are developed and, if possible, sustained.

Sally Robinson, Director of the City of Yonkers Office for the Aging, describes the potential conflicts that could occur when trying to balance the needs of the elderly, city, or other locale, elected officials, and resources stemming from the state, complete with federal and state guidelines that meet the needs of elected officials representing the state and federal government. It is clear that an agency head at the local level is involved in a complex balancing act in order to conduct programs needed by the elderly.

John Wren addresses the political and ideological commitments of the Governor and how these have influenced recent New York State long term care policy developments. The EISEP program is discussed by John Wren at the state level and also by Sally Robinson at the city level. Their different views of the EISEP program illustrate the different balancing processes referred to above.

Ann Cortese describes the dynamics of the policy-making process; she corroborates Abraham Monk's point in a later section about some of the causes of "irrationality" in the policy-making process. Abraham Monk describes both the policy-making process and the course he gives in the Division of Geriatrics and Gerontology on Long Term Care Policy. It is important for students to understand both the policies that currently drive the long term care field, as well as how those policies have been made, are being made and are sustained.

The Municipal Level:
The Case of the City of Yonkers

Sally Robinson

This presentation covers the following issues:

1. Overview of public policies (implicit and explicit) that govern the development and delivery of service at the local/municipal level;
2. Relevance of federal and state policies to the identification of, and response to, need at the local/municipal level; and
3. Needs that are under-addressed by federal and state policies.

OVERVIEW OF PUBLIC POLICIES
(IMPLICIT AND EXPLICIT) THAT GOVERN
THE DEVELOPMENT AND DELIVERY OF SERVICE
AT THE LOCAL/MUNICIPAL LEVEL

What follows is a brief summary of concerns about policy that enables successful service models at the local level. "Successful" means that the models are making a positive difference in what is done, that the policies implemented and developed are enabling of work in response to social need and that such policies are developed where they are absent. "Making a difference" means that they are not doing harm, in addition to doing some good. Some policies are more enabling of a fragmented system than of an integrated, coordinated system, which is viewed as desirable. There are many laws, categorical grant programs and individual entitlements at the federal and state levels that constitute policy stipulating who is going to get what, why they are going to get it, and, in many cases, how agencies should go about making sure they get it. Effort at the local service delivery level focuses on trying to evaluate the relevance of these federal and state policies to local need: that is, to social need identified locally.

The Older Americans Act, a federal policy, is relevant. Yonkers provides a very limited number of services under the Older Americans Act; the city is having more and more of a problem with this particular piece of legislation and the funding generated thereunder, primarily because there seems to be an underlying assumption or presumption that there is something problematic about growing old. It is an age-specific policy; it assumes that if one is a certain age, one is going to need help in certain areas. There is no means test associated with the programs under that act. There are targeting mandates, but in the political context that usually prevails in municipalities at the local level, it is often very difficult to achieve some congruence between the targeting mandates of the Older Americans Act and the electoral quest of local legislators. Yonkers has not necessarily solved this problem; it is doubtful any community has. This is a constraint all communities work under.

Similarly, the New York State Expanded In-Home Services for the Elderly Program (EISEP) has targeted frail elderly, or elderly who are at risk in the community, for services. Here again, under part of that program, there is no means test. Agencies are urged to target their services to special subsets of elderly—frail elderly—who are in need. Thus agencies are caught between the requirements of the law and the policy; the way it is advertised or publicized by legislators, state and local, who are anxious to make the most of this generosity; and by the elderly residents of an area. So it is necessary to work very hard to deliver this service in a way that reaches the targeted population without alienating other groups and their influence on the legislative process. EISEP is a program in which there is some local discretion in terms of organization of the work or organization of the delivery of service. In fact that is true for most programs. In a sense it is the state and federal laws, the guidelines and the descriptions of the grant programs that are very broadly stated in many cases: they are stated in terms of goals. It is up to the localities to come up with objectives to meet those goals and to do it in a way that makes everybody as happy about it as possible in a context of extremely limited funding for elderly services. At times, it would be helpful if federal and state guidelines were more specific.

Another program that is potentially enabling of local models for long term assistance is one in which the New York State Division of Housing and Urban Renewal is beginning to come up with some funding programs to encourage the development of housing options for elderly. This is particularly interesting to municipalities, because it enables promotion of changes in zoning and housing code definitions, which are very important in helping people to manage in the community on a long term basis. If unchanged, these definitions could prevent the development of housing options. For instance there has to be a definition of shared housing in order to work towards a situation where older people can share a house in a one-family neighborhood; and in large cities, where there are concerns about density in neighborhoods, it is taking the state directive which is provided and applying it at the local level; this can be tricky. Property tax exemptions for senior home owners and landlords, which result in rent abatements for certain tenants, is an interesting state policy. The state authorizes localities to exempt certain property owners from property taxes. This is very difficult, particularly for large cities that are struggling with loss of a tax base. And as a local, city office for the aging, Yonkers is caught between knowing that this program is very needed to enable people to stay in their homes in affordable, decent apartments and houses and keeping in mind that the city needs money. The city cannot lose this money; it does not want to provide all these exemptions. Here again it is tricky to follow the state guidelines as far as possible and yet not to the point where the municipality will say, "We're not going to pass a local law to implement this particular policy or entitlement."

To summarize this portion, there are a number of individual statutory entitlements and laws, e.g., the Older Americans Act, that authorize categorical grant programs, some of which may meet local/municipal needs and some of which may not. These federal and state laws contain rules and regulations that inform policy for the funding and delivery of service. In short, they determine who gets what and why and how. However, at times it becomes difficult to balance the needs of local government and clients and state and federal guidelines.

RELEVANCE OF FEDERAL AND STATE POLICIES TO THE IDENTIFICATION OF, AND RESPONSE TO, NEED AT THE LOCAL/MUNICIPAL LEVEL

Fragmented planning units, funding streams and highly bureaucratized implementing authorities are disincentives to collaborative response to multi-problem/need clients who typify the elderly service population. Emphasis on procedure over service outcomes/ results leads to goal displacement and to the inclination of providers to view need as a function of eligibility for benefits which, in turn, influences equitable delivery of service. For example, the ability to "spend down" under Medicaid, rather than service need, often determines access to Medicaid services, especially home care. Further, the ability to pay Medicare deductibles, especially for hospitalization, rather than need for care often determines access to care. Here is just one example of differential treatment of people above income eligibility for Medicaid. The scenario is for two people: one lives in public housing and is paying $80.00 per month for rent, and the other is living in private sector housing and is paying $250.00 per month for rent; their incomes are about the same. They have to spend down $150. The person living in public housing is able to pay for certain medical expenses to the Medicaid eligibility level, and Medicaid will pick up the remainder of his/her costs. The other elder, who is living in private sector housing, cannot afford to spend down—that is, he/she cannot afford to use the money for medical expenses and therefore does not receive the Medicaid benefit. This is becoming more and more common. The issue for the locality is to deal with the problem of age-specific policy, while trying to influence federal and state policies. For instance, at the municipal level, usually there are local recommendations made to state governments, and often to the federal government, in the form of local resolutions; this is an area where service providers can involve themselves. They understand how the programs and policies are working, and they can become involved in that feedback process.

It is necessary to point out that there are variable local capabilities for fiscal support of aging services. More important, it is necessary to note that there is a problem of reaching those most in need with services that are age-specific, rather than need specific. This problem intensifies in a context that reflects increasing prosperity and well-being among the total elderly population. Insufficient attention is being paid to targeting the expanding subgroups of low-income, isolated and chronically-impaired elderly.

A major issue regarding policy that enables successful models of service centers around control or access to service. This is the issue of coordination of service: whether or not there is a single-entry-point model for service. If anything can be done in this fragmented policy context, if there is any successful model that Yonkers is trying to promote, it is a practice model based on an absolute belief in the interdependence of what is done, not only in the aging network, but across systems that affect an older person's life: the legal system, the medical care system, the social care system, the criminal justice system, or any other system. What Yonkers is trying to do is to develop, and this would be an ideal model, mechanisms for inter-system collaboration and coordination under the belief that no system can do its job without the other. In an earlier section, there is a discussion about how geriatrics must become part of the medical school education, and it was noted that doctors are now registering in the school of public health because they realize that in order to care for chronically-ill older people, they must broaden their scope of expertise, understanding and willingness to cooperate. Yonkers is finding that very true in terms of community-based long term care. There was a time when the Yonkers Office on Aging had difficulty getting into area hospitals as a community-based agency in order to participate in discharge planning. Now local hospitals are very anxious to have it come in. The rate of discharge and admissions has gone up with the prospective payment policy under Medicare, so office staff are now welcomed by the medical profession. The staff are helpful in enabling the hospitals to discharge older patients back to the community.

NEEDS THAT ARE UNDER-ADDRESSED
BY FEDERAL AND STATE POLICIES

1. Substantive Support of Informal Caregivers

The needs of family caregivers must be considered. By now, everyone has heard that 80% of social home care received by older people is provided by family, friends and neighbors. Thus the formal delivery of care discussed here is a very small part of the total long term care system in the community. There is no policy that deals adequately with the needs of family caregivers. The New York State Office for the Aging has developed a program to train the trainers of family caregivers. Unfortunately at the local level, there is no staff available or funded under the Older Americans Act or other programs to involve themselves extensively with developing training programs for families and neighbors. This has to be done. This is very important not only in terms of in-kind support and guidance, but in terms of financial support for the efforts of family, for which there is a tremendous need.

2. Empowerment/Autonomy/Self-Determination
Needs, Especially in the Area of Health Care

The elderly often are at the periphery of decision-making about their care and treatment. There are no policies that empower the client to be directly and primarily involved in control of his/her life. There is very little money and there is very little staff to deal with that issue. This is growing more serious as the long term care needs of community aged are becoming more complex. And situations which workers from any system are asked to address are becoming more ambiguous. With the bureaucratization of the delivery system, this very important element in the delivery of service is not being attended to in the way it should. There is too much time pressure on professionals, and there are too many forms to fill out. Thus, the priorities are getting lost.

Self-determination and empowerment are important goals for clients in a highly fragmented policy context that promotes politicization of local response to need, especially if there is a blurring of accountability for effectiveness. Thus, more specificity is needed in federal and state guidelines regarding expected impact. Agency personnel then could work with clients cooperatively to bring about desired outcomes. Again, such agency personnel need to provide feedback to federal and state governments.

In conclusion, the practice model that is going to make a difference in the delivery of long term care services to community elderly will be based on shared beliefs and principles of service that the health care, social care, criminal justice and other systems affecting the elderly are interdependent and can be effective only if there is collaboration and coordination at the local level. This collaboration can be enhanced or impaired by federal and state laws, guidelines, rules and regulations and degree of their responsiveness to local needs.

New York State's Long Term Care Policy and Program Directions

John Wren

This presentation provides background on current New York State long term care policy directions and an illustration of how policy is being implemented, using one program initiative now underway, the EISEP program.

BACKGROUND ON CURRENT NEW YORK STATE LONG TERM CARE POLICY DIRECTIONS

The author has been involved in New York State long term care policy initiatives for about ten years. This work involves activities by a wide variety of agencies at the state level. There is a lot happening in the area, increasingly so over the last five years. Thus, this presentation will just skim the surface by presenting a very general sense of current directions in state policy in this area and also by illustrating the implementation of those policy directions by highlighting just one program initiative, the EISEP program, that is currently under way in the state.

Long term care is a very complex and fragmented system at the state level: there are approximately eight to ten major agencies playing a significant role in this area. One of Governor Cuomo's first actions on taking office was establishment of an interagency body known as the Long Term Care Policy Coordinating Council (LTCPCC). Essentially, this body was designed to bring together the major actors at the state level who are involved in funding long term care programs in order to enhance the coordination of policy development and also to make recommendations to him on what directions he should take as governor. In 1984, the LTCPCC (Lit-

Pic as it is commonly known in state government) sent the Governor a report that provided an overall strategic vision about where the state should be headed in this area. That strategic vision was based upon four major policy principles, which include the following:

1. matching services with actual need;
2. preventing impoverishment;
3. case management; and
4. support for families.

1. Matching Services with Actual Need

Research indicated that there was a need for more non-medical supports. This led to the principle that the State of New York had to do more in the way of having services provided at the community level respond to the actual needs of older people. It is well known that existing services for the most part have been driven by available funding streams, not the needs of older people. Consequently, many services are heavily oriented toward institutional and medical care. It is not that those types of services and care are not important and critically needed; rather, it is that those are the areas that have been developed. However, if one looks at the actual needs of older people, the most pervasive need is for non-medical supports. What makes somebody part of a long term care system is not a medical diagnosis, so much as the ongoing need for support services. Therefore, a tenet of state policy is that more funding and effort has to be directed toward the expansion of non-medical support services.

2. Preventing Impoverishment

A second major principle articulated in the report to the Governor was that older people should not have to impoverish themselves in order to get the care they need. Again, if one looks at the current system, he/she sees that the primary source of payment in this area is Medicaid. Yet elderly persons cannot get help from Medicaid until they first impoverish themselves. And it is known that there are large numbers of people who need services and yet cannot afford to pay for the full cost of those services themselves. Thus there is a problem with using Medicaid as a primary funding source for long term care services. And there is a need to assist elderly people who are not eligible for Medicaid.

3. Case Management

Case management was recognized as another key ingredient for New York State policy to improve system efficiency and client access to services. It was looked at not only from the point of view of providing a mechanism at the local level that would encourage delivery of services in a cost-effective manner, but it was also seen as an important vehicle for increasing the elderly's access to service. The elderly access the long term care system through a variety of different entry points, but mechanisms were needed at the local level to ensure that, regardless of those older people entering the system, there were some uniform procedures for assessing their needs and linking them to needed services.

4. Support for Families

Based on research that documented the important role families play in providing long term care, the fourth key principle in the state policy report was the need to recognize this critical role played by families. Thus, it was essential for the state to begin to revise its policies and programs to complement and support the effort being made by family members. The research references for this point came from the work of Barry Gurland, Ruth Bennett and David Wilder on the issue of informal supports, going back to the cross-national studies they did in the late 1970s. Not only did those studies make a significant contribution to the field of aging in general, but they have had a major impact on public policy formulation at the state level. It is really to their credit, in large measure due to their work, that the principle of helping families is now part of the fabric of state policy. Governor Cuomo accepted the report, endorsed it and essentially directed his Long Term Care Policy Coordinating Council (LTCPCC) to go about the business of developing specific programs and program initiatives that could be used to implement the policy.

THE EISEP PROGRAM AS AN ILLUSTRATION
OF HOW POLICY IS BEING IMPLEMENTED

The Expanded In-Home Services Program for the Elderly (EISEP) was the initiative taken to implement policy. In 1985, LTCPCC recommended to the Governor that he expand the state's provision of case management and in-home services to the elderly through the enhancement of the existing Community Services for the Elderly (CSE) program, which was administered by the State Office for the Aging at the state level, by the Area Agencies on Aging at the county level, and in New York City by the Department for the Aging. Governor Cuomo accepted that proposal and introduced legislation which was approved by the legislature in October, 1986. The law established a uniform program of in-home services to be provided state-wide and targeted at the functionally impaired elderly who are not eligible for Medicaid. A brief review of the service components of the EISEP program shows the link between the program elements and the policy principles mentioned previously. Four types of services can be reimbursed under this program: the first is non-medical, in-home services, including housekeeper, chore and personal care-type services. The second is case management services, including screening, assessment, care planning, eligibility determination, plan implementation, monitoring and follow-up right through to the discharge planning stage. Case management is a requirement for the provision of service under this program: nobody can get services unless he/she goes through the case management process. The third service, non-institutional respite care, refers to forms of respite for family members that may consist of paid patient supervision provided at home or at an adult day care center. EISEP is one of the few home care programs in the country that has a respite care program built into it; this was based on the importance given to the principle to support families. The fourth element is known as ancillary service which essentially allows counties to use up to 10% of their service dollars for unidentified activities about which the state says, "We know that at a clinical level, when a case manager is assessing the needs of older people, there may be something going on in that situation which needs to be addressed and yet there is no specific funding category for it because it doesn't fit under the traditional type of in-home service." It could be the need for architectural barrier removal or the provision of specialized services. Thus, some flexibility has been built into the state program.

In order to receive funding under the EISEP program, counties must put together home care plans, which consist of two components: an assessment of the current home care system in their county, including an overview of the range of home care services currently available, as well as the types of case management currently available in the county; and a plan whereby the county tells the state how it is going to use the EISEP dollars to build on and complement the existing resources available in the community so that those resources are better coordinated and can be accessed better by the elderly.

One special feature of the program is that the state requires counties to use a standardized client assessment tool known as the PATH (Patient Assessment Tool for Home Care). This tool is important for at least two reasons. It was developed by the Renesselaer Polytechnic Institute under a contract with the New York State Departments of Health, Social Services, and the Office for Aging. And it will be the uniform patient assessment tool required by all publicly-aided home care programs in New York State beginning in 1988. All home care programs administered by the Departments of Health and Social Services and the State Office for the Aging will be required to use this tool. It was developed in response to a decade-long demand for a standardized method of assessing the need for home care in this state.

In terms of its current status, the EISEP program is funded this year (1987) at $10.9 million. All but three counties in the state have applied for funding and they are currently going through the agonies and headaches of implementing the new program. 1987-88 is seen as a developmental year for establishment of an infrastructure across the state to improve the provision of non-medical services to the functionally impaired elderly who are not Medicaid-eligible. This will be done in a way that is responsive to their needs. This program also builds a major role for the aging network in the state: to exert its effort and ability in order to influence the way community services are delivered to the elderly across the state.

The Legislative Process with Specific Reference to the County Level

Ann Cortese, MPS

THE REALITIES OF THE LEGISLATIVE PROCESS

The legislative process comes into play at all levels of government, from the town level (sometimes at the hamlet level) right on up to the federal level. This presentation gives some illustrations based on the author's experience as a county office on aging director and then ties these in with the legislative process as it actually occurs at every level. Cliff Whitman, an exceptional director of an area agency in a very progressive county, judging by the standards of other counties in New York State, described the success of the CASA program in Erie County and also mentioned Broome County, whose CASA program was started by Neil Lane. Both programs are working extremely well.

Several years ago, the New York State Department of Social Services (DSS) notified the area agencies that the CASA program would be open to those counties that wanted to enter into it; as head of a county office on aging, the author discussed this option with the county executive, who designated her head of a planning committee to develop a proposal to be presented to the county legislature. The planning committee, consisting of a local DSS representative, the author representing the county office of aging and a representative of the mental health department, labored for nine months on what they believed was a superb proposal. However, the county legislature rejected it. They saw it as another bureaucratic system to be set up. No matter how much the committee stressed the points of central access and central intake, they could not sell the proposal.

The committee was thus obliged to circumvent the system, to

manipulate the system. They developed a code because they found out that some of the other agencies, under state and federal regulations, would not disclose the names of the persons they were serving with the money the county was giving them through its funding mechanism. Thus, they had to develop some kind of system whereby they could get these people into their computer. So they came up with a number system whose chances of being decoded were something like 1 in 3.5 million. The point of this discussion is that this particular item never got to go through the legislative process in the county. That, too, is part of the legislative process. Whoever runs a county agency has to go first to the county executive (or Board of Supervisors, in some counties); at the town level, one goes to the Board of Supervisors or the mayor. Either way, a program can get stopped right there. If it does go further, then one has to go before the proper committee or committees within that process and hope that it gets passed there and then. Of course, then it goes before the full house, the full board, or whatever legislative body the county or town or village is working under. That's just one step in the legislative process.

WORKING WITHIN THE POLITICAL SYSTEM

How does one prepare students to develop successful community services models in a very real political system? One has to research the community, be it a hamlet or county or town. "Research" means more than just gaining knowledge of the services in the community; it also means getting to know the players in the community and developing a feel for the political climate of that political entity. How is this achieved? Taking the time to integrate many factors in the community constitutes a beginning. It was stated earlier that policy makers, academicians and service providers don't speak the same language. In order to be able to work the legislative process in a community, one has to learn to speak many languages.

Service providers are eager to educate the community, other agencies and the legislature about their program, but they have to stop and educate themselves about what is already in existence. They have to learn to speak in the language of the other agencies, so that they can communicate. The key word is planning: do your homework; anticipate the questions; learn the mindset of the powers that be. A good example of this is the author's experience, when soon after she became a county director, the RSVP program was introduced to the legislature. It was turned down three times. It was not introduced through the author's office of aging; it was introduced through a service provider in that county. The introduction was a catastrophe because the persons presenting the program had not done their homework. In retrospect, it was the most embarrassing thing that ever happened to that particular agency. The program did pass eventually, on its fourth introduction to the legislature.

The author's office also had to convince legislators that there was a housing shortage, even though the need was well-known. Invariably, the bottom line is, "How do you know this? Show us." The county office decided that the best way to show it was to do a full-fledged study, and they engaged the services of Columbia University. Dr. David Wilder and several other researchers discovered proof for the powers that be that there was indeed a need for housing. So one has to be creative, almost ingenious, at times, looking for ways to develop needed programs within an already existing system or systems. What is the perfect system? It's the system that works for you. There is no one, perfect long term care system.

INNOVATIVE APPROACHES

The higher one goes into levels of government, the more involved and complicated it gets. The author knew very quickly that there were limitations on funding in the county in which she was working. In the early years it had been fun; money was flowing in, and it was hard to know which programs to put in place first. But after a while, that turned itself around, and it was necessary to look to the future to figure out how to meet known needs with few funds. It was a matter of discovering who could provide services, who was really equipped. As director of a county area agency, the author had to face a fact: they were not equipped to provide a continuum of long term care. There was no way that they could do it. They were getting a thimble-full of money to do an enormous job.

The author began to approach hospitals very boldly. Hospitals were beginning to see the handwriting on the wall—they thought they might be in trouble financially. She approached one hospital about expanding its services out into the community, and the response was, "Oh, we're an acute-care facility; we can't do that kind of thing." And she replied, "Well, why not? Let's take a look at it." They talked, and the hospital's administrators came down to Rockland County. The point is that in order to establish a model program, many different levels within the community and within the state must be dealt with. Before instituting a program called the "Brown Bag Evaluation Clinic," to evaluate the mix of drugs taken by the elderly, the county office on aging had to deal with the New York State Pharmaceutical Society. This, too, is part of the political process.

THE IMPACT OF LEGISLATION

When Governor Cuomo asked the question, "What do you want, SSI or prescription drugs?" he was illustrating how legislation is made and passed. There are always tradeoffs. Every service provider learns this sooner or later. Right now, there is a student in Congressman Gilman's office whom the author is training. The student is going to Washington soon. The student is in shock over the fact that there is no system. At the federal level, providers must deal not only with an aging network, but with all kinds of agencies: the IRS, the State Department, and so on. Legislation comes, in many cases, after the fact. The Congressman's office in which the author works is swamped with calls and cries, most recently from the County Medical Society, because Governor Cuomo passed an administrative law on January 1, 1987 (with no public hearings by the way), that Medicare/Medicaid crossover patients can no longer get the same payment for services they got before. Doctors now either have to pick this up or stop treating these patients. The Congressman's staff had to learn the language of the Medical Society, even though they are not medical people. The physicians also have some legitimate gripes. While it is true that health costs were going out of sight, that situation has been turned around 360 degrees now that so many people are suffering from what has happened as a result of the DRGs and the RUGs.

Right now there is a proposal by the Health Care Financing Administration (HCFA) for a 38% increase in Medicare Part B, primarily because program costs have risen. Currently, payments for the Part B Premium must equal 25% of the program costs, so this increase is going to fall on the backs of the older people. Service providers have to deal with this kind of thing every day. As for the new catastrophic health insurance bill that has delighted so many people and which unquestionably has many good points: who is going to pay for it? This no such thing as a free lunch. Again, that is going to be paid for by the elderly.

In conclusion, service providers must take into consideration many factors in trying to develop a successful model at any level. One cannot escape the fact that the legislative process is tied in with the political process, as well as with all the other factors mentioned earlier in this presentation and by other participants in this conference.

Teaching About U.S. Long Term Care Policies

Abraham Monk, PhD

This section examines two topics: the structural components of federal long term care policies and methods of teaching about federal long term care policy. Basically, the two topics are highly intertwined: it appears that the best way to examine U.S. policy is also the best way to teach about it. This involves using the comparative method, that is, examining U.S. policies by contrasting them with those of other countries. First, policy is examined; then, the course is described. Four aspects, or structural components, of policy listed below are examined within the course as well.

1. POLICY AS A PROCESS

Policy is a dynamic interaction among community factors that leads to some incrementalistic and very often illogical outputs, illogical because they result from the checks and balances between actual objectively-determined needs that are determined by such researchers as David Wilder, but which then have to be confronted with entrenched interests of existing factors in each community. Outcomes are very often, or for the most part, very difficult to predict, as Ann Cortese notes. Policy in the United States is seen as a decentralized, incrementalistic process, and as such, it never really reaches, or it seldom reaches, desired ends. It usually is a compromise between that which is desired and ideologically valued and that which is consented to ultimately by a variety of community forces.

141

2. POLICY AS A PRODUCT

The second level of structural analysis that we develop is policy as a product. In other words, the outcomes of policy which usually are mandates in terms of programs, services and entitlements. While the product aspect is only one facet of policy, almost 80% of the course deals with policy as product, because in the short range, this is what students need to know. And they must know what exactly it is that Medicare or Medicaid pays for and will reimburse under what circumstances: who is eligible and according to what particular formula, depending on what specific diagnostic category they are placed in. Whether it should be that way or not, greater weight must be given to policy as product.

3. POLICY AS IMPACT

The third aspect of policy is policy as impact: the consequences of policy. The course deals with this aspect of policy in regard to the programs that flow from those policies, and their impact in terms of the ripple effect—that is, the systemic consequences of inaugurating a new intervention. Every time one intervenes in a system, one produces consequences in other parts of the system.

4. THE INFRASTRUCTURE OF POLICY

The fourth aspect of policy that is considered is actually the infrastructure of policy, in reference to the ideological foundations, the historical circumstances, the economic realities and the pressures created, or at least the constraints created, by the presence of other programs. The environment in which policy is instituted genuinely affects the nature of the policy that will come out in the process.

THE COURSE ON FEDERAL LONG TERM CARE POLICY

One of the best ways of teaching about policies is by using a comparative method. This means going out of the United States and looking at what is happening in the rest of the world—looking at successful programs in other countries and what we can learn from them. While the focus of the course is not necessarily a comparative one in its totality, a few comparative illustrations are used. The key illustration is one from Canada. Canada has some very advanced and very effective programs of coordinated care and community care case management, particularly in some of the central provinces such as Saskatchewan and Manitoba. But when one looks at the portions of the gross national product spent by Canada and the United States respectively, one sees that the United States spends 30% more, proportionally speaking, of its gross national product on programs in aging. Yet Canada gets better results for less money. The reason the United States over-spends with less effectiveness is that a huge amount of time, which nobody has calculated but which may equal 50% of all actual service delivery expenditures, goes into paper work. This is due to the confrontational nature and suspiciousness that is built into the contractual nature of the service system in the United States.

That is not meant as an indictment of the United States. Nor does it mean that we can adopt the Canadian model — we cannot. It is something nice to look at from a distance, but there is a complexity that emerges from the diseconomy of scale. Basic economics dictates that the larger the scale of the service, the more economies can be built into it. However, this actually works the other way around in this country, the reason being that the larger the scale, the greater the superstructures that are juxtaposed on top of the system to coordinate it. The programs in New York State described by John Wren are good examples. Manitoba has only half a million people; New York State has 20 million. Thus, programs in Manitoba achieve greater visibility: everybody knows who is doing what, and the system thus has built in responsiveness or the responsivity of smaller scale. Up until a few years ago, those of us who taught about policy or programs used to use Denmark as a model. Denmark was an exceptionally beautiful model of a country with the best services for the elderly in the world, and probably they still are. But the entire population of Denmark could fit into just two of the five New York City boroughs — all of Denmark has 4 million people, and all Denmark had to do was develop four or five day care programs, and they resolved the long term care problems in their country. There is an aspect of policy development in the United States that is unique, and therefore we are at a disadvantage in the sense that we can very rarely duplicate or import programs from abroad.

Having reviewed the merits of the comparative approach taken to the study of U.S. long term care policy, let us examine the components of the course on long term care policy given in the Division of Geriatrics and Gerontology. It should be noted that this course is offered only during the summers and really consists of what can be done in the twelve sessions—a considerable challenge since a curriculum like politics is the art of the possible, and the art of the possible is almost impossible in twelve sessions. The course, which is titled "Long Term Care Policy," consists of about six units and is fundamentally a federal policy course with about 80% of its content on federal policy and about 20% on state policy. It begins with an introduction to long term care which includes demographics, the current recipients of long term care, the projections of need, the health status of the aged and the social support systems they have — in other words, the placement of long term care in the social context. The second unit addresses foundations of aging-related policies, looking at aging policies in general, not only the ones on long term care. Students learn about the patterns of policy formation, alluded to above, and review major issues in aging policy that may be current that year. This unit also looks at the scope of federal intervention in the field of aging: the federalism of block grants, revenue sharing, community service block grants, regulatory reforms and so on.

The third unit deals specifically with health care policies: students look at not only the basic provisions of Medicare and Medicaid but also at federal and state relations in long term care, the financing and planning of long term care and the perennial issue of filial responsibility provisions. They also look at how those health care policies really impact on the different service options of long term care: e.g., life care communities, congregate housing, skilled nursing facilities, home health care and so on. The fourth unit deals with proposals for reform and recent reforms in long term care. Long term care is in perpetual fluidity. It is constantly in a state of transformation because consumers are never satisfied or because the system never meets the actual level of need. So students look at reforms in terms of projections of costs of long term care and gatekeeping strategies, which are so popular today, income strategies and community-based strategies. They look at policy options and major initiatives for reform. Then they look at comparative models of long term care. Comparative models may involve comparing the present system with models that may be theoretical, conceptual models developed in the literature or models that are practiced in other countries. This unit also addresses alternatives to institutional care which, by necessity, must be community-based alternatives.

The sixth unit deals with issues of quality control, which is also a reflection of current concerns. Students examine policies aimed at assuring quality control and quality assurance. They also get into issues of impartial mediation, governmental relations, state licensing and federal certifications. This last issue, alluded to by Sally Robinson, is empowerment, that is, the rights of clients and their significant others in terms of advocacy, legislative advocacy, administrative advocacy, litigation and so on. Every effort is made to close the course on a positive note.

One question that should be considered here is, what is the meaning of successful? Presumably, the concept of success is linked to innovativeness. Every time something new is tried, then one can go out and test whether it was successful or not. Innovativeness means experimentation and experimentation is risk-taking. The mid-1980s are not times for risk-taking in service delivery, not because we are incapable of taking or unwilling to take risks, but simply because the policy climate in this country today is not one encouraging of innovation. But we should not despair; this is not the end of the world. From an historical perspective, this country has always gone through peaks and valleys of innovations and constraints or rigidity, the latter being periods in which to consolidate the gains of the periods of innovativeness. At the risk of oversimplifying, some contemporary economists — welfare economists — say that the period from the end of World War II until the late 1960s and early 1970s should be called the age of abundance. It was a period when this country had an optimistic outlook: it seemed that resources were unlimited and that growth would be uninterrupted and would always be on an ascending curve. But the U.S. has entered, particularly after the world oil crises, into a pessimistic mood, into a climate of restraint. That process started during the Carter administration (everything cannot be blamed on Reaganomics). The ten years between 1965-1975 were the most fruitful, most productive, most innovative years for aging that this country has ever known. That period brought us the Older Americans Act; Medicare and Medicaid, with all of their limitations; Supplementary Security Income (SSI); and the indexing of Social Security, which made it into a very forceful social insurance program. This country was, therefore, not only very rich quantitatively in what was produced in those years, but it was able to generate substantial revolutions in policy. SSI, commonly perceived as just a public welfare program, has implicit a very revolutionary policy concept: the safety net concept. The notion that nobody in this society (elderly people primarily, although not only elderly people) can fall below a certain level of income is something new in the history of the U.S. The concept in indexing of Social Security constitutes one of the most effective defenses, in terms of income maintenance, for older persons. But what happened after the mid-1970s? With the Carter Administration came the notion that programs should not be age-specific or age-categorical. The trend initiated then was that programs have to be family-generic. Carter was ideologically committed to the support of the family, a perfectly good idea that resulted in the arrival of Title XX, which was actually very ineffectual for the most part, or at least it was not focused on the promotion of programs for the elderly. This leads to the conclusion that this country now is in a period of declining innovativeness, mostly because of cost containment and restrictiveness, which place limits on innovativeness as well as on the criteria for success. Right now the criterion by which success is judged is not how good the program is for the older recipient, but how much money it is going to save. If anything, current policies dictate that the success of programs be measured by the mini-max concept: minimum cost and maximum gain. There is a positive quality in that, but not much. Even if reality is not very encouraging, long term care educators must not, when they are looking at success, lose their ability to communicate to their students the notion that this country must persist in the development of new models of services, to be more creative than ever. And if courses in the Division of Geriatrics and Gerontology, particularly the course in policy, contributes to that, this program will make a substantial social contribution.

PART IV:
CONCLUSIONS

Concluding Remarks and Suggested Issues for Further Discussion

Ruth Bennett, PhD
Eloise H. P. Killeffer, EdM

Counties, towns and hamlets, like cities, states and societies, are not impervious to the social climates or cultural milieux within which they find themselves. These cultural climates inform the policies and practices which trickle down to local communities. Thus, planners of policies and programs must assess the social climate at any given time when undertaking these activities.

At present, there is a cost-cutting mentality afoot, which has been noted by a number of contributors to these proceedings. Thus, this may be the time for local communities to think about developing indigenous ways of providing community-based long term care services and programs for the elderly. It seems obvious at this time that those most concerned with providing the best care and services possible to their elderly are families and the communities in which the elderly reside. Ultimately, the buck stops there. But if families and communities truly believe their elders deserve the best possible care, they will have to organize themselves to secure it.

As so many of the papers contained in this volume indicate, federal, state and other public funding sources go only so far and no further: either they restrict benefits and entitlements to certain groups or they provide limited funding to all groups of the elderly. It then becomes a challenge to the resourcefulness and skills of the administrators of agencies and other community leaders to use these funds most efficiently and effectively and, frequently, to raise additional funds in order to provide very high quality services. If these agencies are fortunate enough to be located in resource-rich and caring communities, their fund-raising efforts may be well-rewarded. If, however, they are not, they may become frustrated and, perhaps, discouraged. Thus, many administrators and community leaders are confronted with the daunting tasks of organizing available resources and locating them when they are not obvious. In the end, however, talented community-based service or program administrators must take stock of what they have to work with and move on from there.

The successful administrator must be cognizant to some degree of several factors in order to enlist the aid of potential allies in the community: the condition and position of the elderly within the community; the degree to which ageism in all its many forms permeates a community; the degree of gerontological awareness or education within a community; and the identification of, and availability of, potential resources within a community. These issues are addressed below.

THE CONDITION AND POSITION OF THE ELDERLY WITHIN THE COMMUNITY

There are several reasons why the current cohort of old people has had little say over the course of their lives at the end. Isolation, feminization of aging and frailty are but three.

Isolation: Many aged are socially isolated from the mainstream of society rather than socially integrated: as of 1987, 8 million of 28 million lived alone; most of the rest lived with elderly spouses and may constitute isolated pairs. Five percent were segregated in institutions and no one knows just how many were ghettoized in segregated housing or communities for the elderly. Such isolation or segregation may mean that they can exert very little influence over states of societal consensus. They are often isolated due to factors beyond their control (e.g., frailty, forced retirement from the labor force, gender, lack of education, illness, personality traits and fearfulness). In many ways, what happens to the aged is similar to what happens to minority groups and other powerless groups. There is always a question about what they will do. Will they further segregate or ghettoize themselves, isolate themselves individually, work only with other elderly or seek allies with whom to work and work out compromises? These are tough decisions and processes. Insofar as all of us will be elderly, we can and should influence the isolation-integration process. In some countries (e.g., Sweden, Holland, West Germany) the elderly are integrated into the mainstream by policy.

Feminization of Aging: Most of the aged (2/3 of those over 65; 3/4 of those over 75) are women and that reduces their capacity to influence states of consensus. Their natural allies may be their caregivers (i.e., middle-aged women) but they too may have very little influence over states of consensus. This may be true worldwide. Few women are leaders of women. Many women have resources but do not control their use, so they cannot advocate for the elderly as well as their numbers might suggest. The Older Women's League (OWL) and other older womens' groups are trying to change this in the United States.

Frailty and Other Vulnerabilities: Many aged are poor, frail and depressed. These conditions also may keep them from working, lobbying and advocating on their own behalf.

THE DEGREE OF AGEISM IN A COMMUNITY

Ageism is a factor working against the elderly; many elderly feel as if they are invisible. Reducing ageism requires massive efforts in prejudice reduction, which may happen as more people realize they too will grow older. But ageism is a real and hard-to-change part of our youth-oriented cultural climate. Compounding ageism per se are other cultural themes not unrelated to ageism: cost-cutting and/ or tax-cutting and the medicalization of many human services, which may increase their cost to society and certainly de-emphasizes all but the medical aspects of aging.

These cultural themes cannot be changed easily and it is probably necessary to learn how to live with them and to work with and/or around them. In any given community, there may be individuals who adhere to the cost-cutting and medicalization viewpoints and who are trying to frame the demographic imperative issues in those terms. But there are alternatives: citizens in West Germany, Sweden, Canada, Holland and Australia, for example, support policies based on the position that the elderly gave them the societies they live in today (both the good and bad aspects) and they therefore owe it to the elderly to honor and care for them.

THE DEGREE OF GERONTOLOGICAL AWARENESS OR EDUCATION IN A COMMUNITY

Very little attention has been paid to the positive side of aging, to the benefits, to what the aged bring to a family or the community in which they reside. Much more research and thinking is needed to determine the positive contributions made by the elderly. It is difficult to cite a single U.S. study about this, even including the few studies of grandparenting that have been done. In contrast, studies about costs proliferate. This lack of awareness about the benefits of an aging society may contribute to the general lack of awareness about aging issues.

Few communities seem conscious of the fact that the bulk of caregiving is done by middle-aged daughters who seem to be "sandwiched" between two sets of conflicting, but equally salient, role expectations. Should they use their scarce resources and time to support their children or their several sets of aging parents (and, perhaps, grandparents)? While they are being tormented by these conflicts, middle-aged women are being encouraged, sometimes forced, to go back to work or school. It is no wonder that middle-age crises are so prevalent. Can these crises be resolved by each person individually, one at a time, or do they cry out for social solutions? Pluralistic ignorance has no justification in such a tension-laden arena. There is much policy talk now about "returning" the care of the aged to families, of family supports, informal supports, natural support networks and replacing the formal service system. It is hard to see how demographics, the social climate and the cultural picture can lend themselves to strengthening informal or family supports.

Demographics: There is at present a declining birth rate and an increasing number of old people, with the greatest growth in the sector over age 75. This means there are fewer younger people available for caring for elders as well as for working. According to Callahan (1987), between 1980 and 2040, there will be a 41% increase in this country's population and a 160% increase in those 65 and older. In fact, more women will be needed in the labor force to compensate for the drop in birth rate and will not be available for caretaker roles. Census data up to 1986 indicate there has been a significant increase in women in the labor force: 51.1 million in 1985, or 2.5 times the number in 1950. Further, 50% of all women age 16 and older were either working or looking for work in 1985, compared with only one-third in 1950. Therefore, the job of caring for the elderly will have to be shared by everyone.

Social Climate: The current social climate encourages women to work; indeed, there are very few intact nuclear families, let alone extended families. The job comes first: geographic and social mobility are highly valued even by those old persons abandoned as their children move out or up.

Cultural Picture: As noted above, this consists of negative stereotyping, including viewing the aged as nonproductive by young and other elderly alike. Thus there is little motivation to consider their problems to be of high priority.

Despite these factors, many studies have found that most caretaking is done by relatives and that many families plan to provide care up to the point where they are stressed by the deteriorating condition of the older person. Many families and non-related caretakers shoulder immense burdens for as long as they can. Often they decide to institutionalize because there are no alternatives. In theory, a well-worked out alternative service delivery system, including home care, day care, transportation, respite care and a variety of non-traditional services should allow more families to keep older persons at home. These services were described in the preceding chapters and, as many of the authors indicated, it is difficult to obtain funds to provide them. As several federally-funded studies have shown, community service use does not reduce costs, even with the most sophisticated kinds of case management. Therefore, there has been little incentive to replicate such non-traditional services at the taxpayers' expense.

However, changes in the types and manner of long term care service delivery and other lifestyle options for the elderly probably will occur if only because of education. At present, the most educated cohort is entering the old age group—the group that was age 17 in 1939-1940, half of whom graduated from high school, a dramatic increase over 17-year-olds in earlier periods. This group may make greater demands for services and will probably use them. Moreover, they may demand improvements in the quality of life in general. This will not be without great cost. But in a caring community, costs are not a major issue. Such communities have found, and will continue to find, ways and means of caring for their elders and they will serve as models for other communities seeking to do likewise. However, in order to provide care for these elders, agency directors and community leaders will have to work together.

To prevent intergenerational polarization, communities may have to work harder to integrate the elderly. Practically, this may mean using as examples lifestyles developed in other westernized countries such as Canada, England, Sweden and France. These countries seem to have learned a bit more than the United States about how to shore up natural or informal systems such as communities, parishes and families; whereas the U.S. still seems to be in the business of inventing ways to fragment, rather than support, these informal systems. This country must rethink its policies so as to reward, rather than beggar, caring communities.

No community can any longer afford to think of the elderly as "them versus us." This revision in thinking requires that a great deal of information be available to politicians, professionals and laypersons alike: political and social decisions cannot continue to be made for each age group separately as if each exists in a vacuum. Since it is now known that 70% of all persons born today are expected to grow old, decision-making at all levels should expand to include lifestyle choices and options that make sense over the lifespan.

More lifestyle options should be available that can be sustained or tolerated by the community for a lifetime. For example, in some communities, zoning laws need to be changed to allow unrelated elders to share homes. People need support, help and education at all ages. The helping process should not be seen as stopping at age 18 and resuming again at age 65. Not everyone can be counted on to build a resource network to last a lifetime; many networks may be fragile throughout the lifespan and may need regular shoring up. One is not a failure at age 45 if a fragile network falls apart. Networks do fall apart, and for all sorts of reasons. For instance, the average age of widowhood in the U.S. is 56. Therefore, communities, societies and other political and social entities are worthless if people of all ages and stages within them cannot count on support and sustenance with dignity.

Learning how to be an old person may be something each person has to do quite early in life, and it may not come naturally at this point in our history, especially when few people have role models of successful aging. Aging on a large scale is a new phenomenon on the world scene. The point is that everyone may need to learn about aging and the aged in order to live with the process: aging is here to stay and it certainly beats the alternative.

Several groups in the community are particularly in need of learning about aging immediately: *the elderly themselves*, who seem to be having a difficult time of it, based on research on depression, suicide (25% of all suicides are elderly, even though they are but 12% of the population), demoralization and related attitudes; *grandparents and grandchildren*, whom research shows are virtually non-interactive; *young families*, whose relationships might improve if elders were involved but who know precious little about how to re-create extended families; *neighbors*, who could be friendly visitors, if they but knew how; *politicians and policymakers*, whose decisions affect everyone; and *professionals* in all the helping professions.

More and more old people with, or even without, resources may be so discouraged by intergenerational tensions that they may continue to segregate themselves into old-age ghettos such as retirement communities, just to escape the fray. This may represent a great loss to each community, the overall effects of which have not as yet been felt or which are just beginning to be felt. Despite persistent survey results showing that morale is highest among the elderly in age-segregated (as opposed to age-integrated) settings, the implications of these findings must be considered: can any segregation be good? This country has just emerged from century-long battles to desegregate the races and genders. Will it take another battle to desegregate the generations?

Age divisions may well replace class divisions on the political and social scenes permanently unless there is a conscious effort to stop the process. Old people may not wish to support schools with their taxes; young people may not wish to support Social Security. Against a backdrop of ageism, it is not hard to tell who will win. However, as the aged cohorts grow increasingly numerous and better educated, they will constitute a mighty political and social force. Society will not be able to ignore them, as it often does children, because most of the elderly vote.

IDENTIFICATION OF POTENTIAL AND AVAILABLE RESOURCES WITHIN A COMMUNITY

It is clear that cultural themes must be changed quickly in order for everyone to change his/her attitudes and to adjust to societal aging. Caring is something people in this country do quite naturally; the notion needs only to be extended to cover the lifespan, to learn how to promote and encourage intergenerational friendships. New professions of a caring nature will arise that will require humanistic and interdisciplinary skills (e.g., case managers, case coordinators, long term care planners and counselors for extended families). At this time, cost-benefit research seems to be in vogue. It is known that an aging population will be costly, but the benefits are as yet unclear. However, a different approach to service and research is needed. Answers would be forthcoming if more humanistic studies were conducted, yet the trend against humanistic research continues. But within any given community, such studies will have to be done in order to determine who needs services of what kinds. The social climate, the attitudes of community residents, the degree of willingness to come forward to assist the elderly, the means available for doing so — all must be assessed. This kind of investigation will have to go beyond the standard needs assessment inventories, especially since these are usually focused on the elderly. The needs and resources of entire communities, however their boundaries are determined, will have to be assessed in order to deliver high quality community-based services. Everyone should be intent on encouraging and conducting such research, on the assumption that what is discovered to be good for the elderly will, ultimately, be good for us all.

CONCLUSIONS

Aging is a burning issue because of worldwide demographics. This is called by gerontologists the "demographic imperative." Throughout the world, the aged (65 and over) population is the fastest-growing, and of those, the 85 and over group is fastest of all. The very old and frail can be kept alive longer than ever before.

While these data sound very positive, they have many implications, not the least of which are the costs to society. This has become a hot political issue in the U.S. and elsewhere and has led also to "graybashing" in the media and elsewhere. The major implication of the demographic imperative seems to be the need to change our cultural themes and values. While caring is something done very naturally in most families, this society must become more caring in general and must extend the notion of caring to cover the lifespan. At this point, the United States seems to be more concerned about the costs of caring than the structures for, and processes of, caring. The aged population is viewed as a threat rather than a source of pride, as a disproportionate consumer of public funds rather than as a remarkable testament to the achievements of a highly sophisticated society. Furthermore, this society has not addressed the benefits of an aging population. It is imperative that this country give some thought to changing from a youth-oriented to a person-oriented society.

It seems easier to address these issues at the community level than at a societal level and to develop community-based services at that level. If each community were to concentrate on caring for its elders, using public monies sensibly where needed, especially to assist those who somehow fall between the cracks (as done by many of this volume's authors, who are agency workers and directors), the development of community-based services would be speeded up significantly and the goal of developing caring communities might seem more achievable. For these reasons, the faculty of the Division of Geriatrics and Gerontology wanted their students in long term care administration to attend this conference, at which community agency directors and leaders described the ways and means used to organize and operate their services on behalf of the community elderly.

APPENDICES

RECOMMENDED READINGS

Abramovice, B., *Long Term Care Administration.* New York, NY: The Haworth Press, 1987.

Bennett, R., Frisch, S., Gurland, B. & Wilder, D. (eds.), *Coordinated Service Delivery Systems for the Elderly.* New York, NY: The Haworth Press, 1984.

Callahan, D., *Setting Limits: Medical Goals in an Aging Society.* New York, NY: Simon & Schuster, 1987.

Center for Policy Research, National Governors' Association, *Building Affordable Long Term Care Alternatives: Integrating State Policy.* Washington, DC: National Governors' Association, April 1987.

Hughes, S. L., *Long-Term Care Options in an Expanding Market.* Homewood, IL: Dow Jones-Irwin, 1986.

Morrison, I., Bennett, R., Frisch, S. & Gurland, B., (eds.), *Continuing Care Retirement Communities: Political, Social, and Financial Issues.* New York, NY: The Haworth Press, 1985.

National Institute on Adult Day Care, *Standards for Adult Day Care.* Washington, DC: The National Council on the Aging, Inc., 1984.

National League for Nursing, *Community-Based Initiatives in Long Term Care.* Pub. No. 20-2153. New York, NY: National League for Nursing, 1986.

New York State Office for the Aging, *Community Services for the Elderly: An Assessment of Program Effectiveness.* Albany, NY: New York State Office for the Aging, no date.

Padula, H., *Developing Adult Day Care: An Approach to Maintain-*

ing Independence for Impaired Older Persons. Washington, DC: The National Council on the Aging, Inc., 1986.

Rabin, D. L. and Stockton, P., *Long-Term Care for the Elderly: A Factbook.* New York, NY: Oxford University Press, 1987.

U.S. Department of Health & Human Services, *The Evaluation of the National Long Term Care Demonstration: Final Report.* Prepared by Mathematica Policy Research Inc., Princeton, NJ, 1986.

Zawadski, R. T., *Community-Based Systems of Long Term Care.* New York, NY: The Haworth Press, 1984.

THE EISEP (EXAPANDED IN-HOME SERVICES FOR THE ELDERLY PROGRAM) SCREENING INSTRUMENT

Section O. Service Plan Summary

1 Date: _____ **2** Prepared by: _____

3 Client Name: _____ **4** Client ID: _____ **5** Telephone ( ) _____

6 Address: _____

7 Problems

Desired Outcome/Goal
_____
_____
_____

8 Services

Service Type	Code	Days Week	Visits Week	Hours Week	Start Date	Estimated Cost	Provider

9 Total Service cost: $ _____

Medication cost: $ _____

Equipment cost: $ _____

Physician visits: $ _____

TOTAL: $ _____

159

The EISEP Screening Instrument (continued)

10 Referral to *Check all that apply.*

☐ Hospital   ☐ Nursing Home   ☐ CHHA   ☐ AAA   ☐ Discharge (Reason) _____

☐ Adult Home   ☐ LTHHCP   ☐ Personal Care   ☐ Other *Specify:* _____

11 **Next assessment in:**

☐ 30   ☐ 60   ☐ 90   ☐ 120   ☐ 6

Days   Days   Days   Days   Mos.

FOOTNOTES

1. The screening instrument from which this is excerpted is the initial, early version currently being used by the New York State Office for the Aging (SOFA) in implementing the Expanded In-Home Services for the Elderly Program (EISEP). SOFA and the Departments of Health and Social Services are still working on a standardized instrument for assessing clients for in-home attendant programs, based on the first 2 1/2 years of program experience.

2. SOFA requires programs participating in EISEP to use this instrument to determine eligibility. However, local programs are free to augment this screen with their own questions, subject to review by SOFA.

3. For further information, contact Marcus Harazin, Director, Expanded In-Home Services for the Elderly Program, New York State Office for the Aging, 2 Empire State Plaza, Albany, New York, 12223; (518) 474-8147.

CONFERENCE SPEAKERS

Ruth Bennett, PhD
Director of Graduate Studies
Division of Geriatrics and Gerontology
Columbia University School of Public Health
Tower 3, 29-F, 100 Haven Avenue
New York, New York 10032

Ellen Camerieri, CSW
Executive Director
Riverdale Senior Services, Inc.
2600 Netherland Avenue
Bronx, New York 10463

Ann Cortese, MPS
District Manager
Office of Congressman Benjamin Gilman
223 Route 59
Monsey, New York 10951

Lucien Cote, MD
Associate Professor of Neurology
   and Rehabilitation Medicine
College of Physicians & Surgeons
Columbia University
630 West 168th Street
New York, New York 10032

K. Della Ferguson, PhD
Associate Professor of Psychology
Institute of Gerontology
Utica College of Syracuse University
Burrstone Road
Utica, New York 13502

Susana Frisch, MA
Program Coordinator
Division of Geriatrics and Gerontology
Columbia University

School of Public Health
Tower 3, 29-F, 100 Haven Avenue
New York, New York 10032

Lois Grau, PhD
Associate Director
Brookdale Research Institute
Fordham University
113 West 60th Street
New York, New York 10023

Barry Gurland, MD
Head
Division of Geriatrics and Gerontology
Columbia University
School of Public Health
Tower 3, 30-F, 100 Haven Avenue
New York, New York 10032

Ralph E. Hall, MA
Executive Vice President
Morningside House
1000 Pelham Parkway South
Bronx, New York 10461

Douglas Holmes, PhD
President, Community Research Applications
    and Director of Research
Hebrew Home for the Aged at Riverdale
5901 Palisade Avenue
Bronx, New York 10471

Igal Jellinek
Executive Director
Council of Senior Centers
    and Services of New York City, Inc.
275 Seventh Avenue
New York, New York 10001

George Kaplan
Director of Home Care Services
Jewish Association of Services
  for the Aged (JASA)
40 West 68th Street
New York, New York 10023

Eloise H. P. Killeffer, EdM
Practicum Coordinator
  and Division Administrator
Division of Geriatrics and Gerontology
Columbia University
School of Public Health
Tower 3, 29-F, 100 Haven Avenue
New York, New York 10032

Theresa L. Martico-Greenfield, MPH
Special Assistant to the Executive Vice President
Jewish Home & Hospital for Aged
120 West 106th Street
New York, New York 10025

Abraham Monk, PhD
Professor
School of Social Work
Columbia University
804 McVickar Hall
622 West 113th Street
New York, New York 10027

Sally Robinson
Director
Yonkers Office for the Aging
201 Palisade Avenue
Yonkers, New York 10703

Shura Saul, EdD, ACSW
Educational Coordinator
Kingsbridge Heights Manor

3426 Cannon Place
Bronx, New York 10463

Lynn Tepper, EdD
Assistant Clinical Professor
Columbia University
School of Dental and Oral Surgery
630 West 168th Street
New York, New York 10032

John Toner, EdD
Assistant Professor of Clinical Public Health
Division of Geriatrics and Gerontology
Columbia University
School of Public Health
Tower 3, 30-F, 100 Haven Avenue
New York, New York 10032

Clifford Whitman, MSW
Commissioner
Erie County Department of Senior Services
Erie County Office Building Room 1329
95 Franklin Street
Buffalo, New York 14202-3968

David Wilder, PhD
Deputy Director
Center for Geriatrics and Gerontology
Columbia University and New York State
    Office of Mental Health
Tower 3, 30-F, 100 Haven Avenue
New York, New York 10032

John Wren
Assistant Director for Program
    Development and Evaluation
New York State Office for the Aging
2 Empire State Plaza
Albany, New York 12223

COLUMBIA UNIVERSITY SCHOOL OF PUBLIC HEALTH DIVISION OF GERIATRICS AND GERONTOLOGY ADVISORY COMMITTEE DIRECTORY

Barry Gurland, MD, Chair

John Barsa, MD
Assistant Clinical Professor
Department of Psychiatry
College of Physicians & Surgeons
Columbia University

Ruth Bennett, PhD
Director of Graduate Studies
Division of Geriatrics & Gerontology
Columbia University
School of Public Health
Tower 3, 29-F, 100 Haven Avenue
New York, New York 10032

Ellen Camerieri, CSW
Executive Director
Riverdale Senior Services, Inc.
2600 Netherland Avenue
Bronx, New York 10463

William Connelly
Group Business Director
Mental Health & Aging
Pharmaceutical Division
Sandoz Inc.
59 Route 10
East Hanover, New Jersey 07936

Stanley Cortell, MD
Professor of Clinical Medicine
Division of Nephrology
St. Luke's-Roosevelt Hospital
Amsterdam Avenue & 114th Street
New York, New York 10025

Ann Cortese, MPS
District Manager for Congressman Benjamin Gilman
223 Route 59
Monsey, New York 10951

Lucien J. Cote, MD
Associate Professor of Neurology
  & Rehabilitation Medicine
College of Physicians & Surgeons
Columbia University
630 West 168th Street
New York, New York 10032

Thomas F. Coughlin
Executive Vice President and Administrator
Isabella Geriatric Center
515 Audubon Avenue
New York, New York 10040

Margaret E. Donnelly, PhD
Associate Professor of Sociology
Herbert H. Lehman College, CUNY
Bedford Park Boulevard West
Bronx, New York 10468-1589

K. Della Ferguson, PhD
Associate Professor of Psychology
Institute of Gerontology
Utica College of Syracuse University
Burrstone Road
Utica, New York 13502

Saul Freedman, PhD
Director of National Consultants
American Foundation for the Blind
15 West 16th Street
New York, New York 10011

Susana Frisch, MA
Curriculum Coordinator and Program Administrator

Division of Geriatrics & Gerontology
Columbia University
School of Public Health
Tower 3, 29-F, 100 Haven Avenue
New York, New York 10032

Lois Grau, PhD
Associate Director
Brookdale Research Institute
Fordham University
113 West 60th Street
New York, New York 10032

Barry Gurland, MD
Head
Division of Geriatrics & Gerontology
Columbia University
School of Public Health
Tower 3, 30-F, 100 Haven Avenue
New York, New York 10032

Ralph E. Hall, MA
Executive Vice President
Morningside House
1000 Pelham Parkway South
Bronx, New York 10461

Theresa H. Hauber, MPH
Professional Education Coordinator
Transplant Foundation of New Jersey
65 East Northfield Road
Livingston, New Jersey 07039

Douglas Holmes, PhD
President, Community Research Applications
   and Director of Research
Hebrew Home for the Aged at Riverdale
5901 Palisade Avenue
Bronx, New York 10471

Peter R. Holt, MD
Professor of Medicine
St. Luke's-Roosevelt Hospital, S & R 12
Amsterdam Avenue & 114th Street
New York, New York 10025

Ann Hudis, MPH, EdD
Professor
112 Locust Lane
Irvington-on-Hudson, New York 10533

Igal Jellinek
Executive Director
Council of Senior Centers & Services
   of New York City, Inc.
275 Seventh Avenue
New York, New York 10001

Daphne Joslin, PhD, MPH
Long Term Care Planning Specialist
Office of Long Term Care Planning & Policy
New York City Department for the Aging
2 Lafayette Street
New York, New York 10007

Lucie S. Kelly, RN, PhD, FAAN
Professor of Public Health & Nursing and Head,
   Division of Health Administration
Columbia University
School of Public Health
600 West 168th Street
New York, New York 10032

Jennifer Kelsey, PhD,
Professor and Head
Division of Epidemiology
Columbia University
School of Public Health

Tower 2, 30-D, 100 Haven Avenue
New York, New York 10032

Eloise H. P. Killeffer, EdM
Practicum Coordinator
Division of Geriatrics & Gerontology
Columbia University
School of Public Health
Tower 3, 29-F, 100 Haven Avenue
New York, New York 10032

Robert A. Killeffer, CBC
Marketing Communications
141 Oak Street
New Canaan, Connecticut 06840

Corinne Kirschner, MPhil.
Director of Social Research
American Foundation for the Blind
15 West 16th Street
New York, New York 10011

Donald S. Kornfeld, MD
Professor of Clinical Psychiatry
Columbia University College of Physicians & Surgeons
630 West 168th Street
New York, New York 10032

Joseph Krevisky
Manager of Management & Supervisory Training
Office of Staff Development & Training
Human Resources Administration
FAS Bureau of Management Systems
60 Hudson Street, 9th Floor, Room 9438
New York, New York 10013

Rafael Lantigua, MD
Assistant Professor of Clinical Medicine
AIM Clinic

Vanderbilt Clinic 2-205
Presbyterian Hospital
610 West 168th Street
New York, New York 10032

Eugene Litwak, PhD, Professor and Head,
Division of Sociomedical Sciences
Columbia University
School of Public Health
600 West 168th Street
New York, New York 10032

Theresa L. Martico-Greenfield, MPH
Special Assistant to the Executive Vice President
Jewish Home & Hospital for Aged
120 West 106th Street
New York, New York 10025

Patricia A. Miller, MEd, OTR
Assistant Professor in Clinical Occupational Therapy
Programs in Occupational Therapy
Columbia University
630 West 168th Street
New York, New York 10032

Esther Mishkin, MSW
Director
Selfhelp Community Services
Washington Heights Office
717 West 177th Street
New York, New York 10033

Abraham Monk, PhD
Professor
School of Social Work
Columbia University
804 McVickar Hall
622 West 113th Street
New York, New York 10025

Ian Morrison, EdD
President
Greer Woodycrest
RR 2, Box 1000
Millbrook, New York 12454

Mary Mundinger, DrPH
Dean
School of Nursing
Columbia University
617 West 168th Street
New York, New York 10032

Lloyd Nurick, CAE
Executive Director
New York State Association of Homes & Services
   for the Aging
194 Washington Avenue, 4th Floor
Albany, New York 12210

Nicholas Rango, MD
Associate Professor of Health & Society
Barnard College
3009 Broadway
New York, New York 10025

Sally Robinson
Director
Yonkers Office for the Aging
201 Palisade Avenue
Yonkers, New York 10703

S. Jaime Rosovski, PhD
450 West End Avenue #7C
New York, New York 10024

Joseph J. Ryan, MD
Medical Director
Center for Geriatric Care
Morristown Memorial Hospital

95 Mt. Kemble Avenue
Morristown, New Jersey 07960

Shura Saul, EdD, ACSW
Educational Coordinator
Kingsbridge Heights Manor
3426 Cannon Place
Bronx, New York 10463

Marilyn Shilkoff, EdD
Aging Research Services
25 Larchmont Avenue
Larchmont, New York 10538

Barbara Silverstone, DSW
Executive Director
The Lighthouse-New York State Association
   for the Blind
111 East 59th Street
New York, New York 10022

David Soyer, MSSW
Director of Community Services
Jewish Association of Services for the Aged (JASA)
40 West 68th Street
New York, New York 10023

Lynn Tepper, EdD
Assistant Clinical Professor and Director
Division of Behavioral Science
School of Dental & Oral Surgery
Columbia University
630 West 168th Street
New York, New York 10032

Jeanne Teresi, PhD
Center for Geriatrics & Gerontology
Columbia University
Tower 3, 29-F, 100 Haven Avenue
New York, New York 10032

Bonnie Teschendorf, PT, MHA
Assistant Professor
Program in Physical Therapy
Columbia University
630 West 168th Street
New York, New York 10032

John Toner, EdD
Assistant Professor
Division of Geriatrics & Gerontology
Columbia University School of Public Health
Tower 3, 30-F, 100 Haven Avenue
New York, New York 10032

Bruce Vladeck, PhD
President
United Hospital Fund
55 Fifth Avenue
New York, New York 10003-4392

Jane Weiler, CSW
Director
Fort Washington Houses Senior Center
99 Fort Washington Avenue
New York, New York 10032

Clifford Whitman, MSW
Commissioner
Erie County Department of Senior Services
Erie County Office Building, Room 1329
95 Franklin Street
Buffalo, New York 14202-3968

David Wilder, PhD
Deputy Director
Center for Geriatrics & Gerontology
Columbia University
Tower 3, 30-F, 100 Haven Avenue
New York, New York 10032

Michael Wilkes, Jr., MD
Public Health Officer
New York City Department of Health
125 Worth Street, Box 12
New York, New York 10013

Milton Keynes UK
Ingram Content Group UK Ltd.
UKHW031134141024
449569UK00006B/191